Health Care for the Poor and Elderly: Meeting the Challenge

Health Care for the Poor and Elderly: Meeting the Challenge

Based on the Seventh Private Sector Conference, 1982

Edited by Duncan Yaggy

Foreword by William G. Anlyan

Duke Press Policy Studies
Duke University Press
Durham, North Carolina   1984

Library of Congress Cataloging in Publication Data

Main entry under title:

Health care for the poor and elderly.

(Duke Press policy studies)
Includes index.
1. Aged—Medical care—United States—Congresses.
2. Poor—Medical care—United States—Congresses.
3. Medicare—Congresses. 4. Medicaid—Congresses.
I. Yaggy, Duncan. II. Series. [DNLM: 1. Health Services—
United States—Congresses. 2. Health Services for the
Aged—United States—Congresses. 3. Medical indigency—
United States—Congresses. W3 PR945F 7th 1982h /
WT 30 P961 1982h]

ISBN 0-8223-0508-9

Contents

Tables and Figures

Tables

Figures

Foreword

From this remove it is difficult to recapture the confidence and optimism of 1965. It is hard to remember that government was then thought to be a constructive and creative force, capable of righting wrongs and solving problems. It is hard to imagine that Medicaid, Medicare, and the war in Vietnam were all launched in that same year—without a tax increase because their costs would be kept under control! It is easy to understand why our confidence in government has diminished in the years since.

The Private Sector Conferences at Duke University started in 1977, when it seemed important to respond to a government apparently determined to restructure our system of health care. In 1977 the private sector was on the defensive, and the conference was filled with protest and complaint. Subsequent conferences have displayed a more thoughtful and positive outlook.

This year marks a turning point. We convene as the public sector retreats. Public hospitals and clinics are being reduced or closed. Government support for health care services to the poor and elderly has been cut, but deficits loom and further reductions are now in prospect. Reluctant to go on record as supporting the elimination of needed services or the disqualification of needy people, governments have simply reduced their payments to providers. Medicare and Medicaid never paid full cost, but they formerly paid a lesser amount, called "allowable cost." Now they pay a diminishing share of allowable cost and leave physicians and hospitals to figure out how services to the poor and the elderly—and those without coverage of any kind—are to be continued and financed.

Can the private sector meet this challenge? The answer is unclear, but two things are certain: First, the problem is growing, for people over sixty-five make up the fastest growing segment of our population. Second, the traditional remedy will not suffice. Many providers serving large numbers of Medicare and Medicaid patients—particularly urban teaching hospitals—are finding that cost shifting is no longer workable. The cost to be shifted is too large, and the number of charge-paying patients is too small. For their part, employers and insurers protest against the growing burden of the costs they are asked to assume, and they are seeking ways to reduce it.

What can be done? The options are limited. To reduce the cost of services to the poor and the elderly, society must reduce the number of those eligible, limit the services which they are provided, substitute less expensive for more expensive services, or cut their cost through changes in organization, delivery, or financing.

The Seventh Private Sector Conference assembled physicians, economists, hospital administrators, planners, educators, and policy makers to debate these options for a day and a half. Their discussion exposed sharp differences of opinion and raised fundamental questions:

Does our society spend enough on health care services for its poor and elderly?

Do we buy the right services? In the right proportions?

Do we spend too much on nursing home services? Should we find less expensive, less impersonal ways of caring for the elderly?

Do we spend enough on health promotion and disease prevention?

Do we spend too much on medical and hospital services to the dying?

Who are the poor who cannot afford health care services? What services do they need most?

Should all the elderly be eligible for Medicare services, or should a means test be imposed?

Can we protect access to health care services for the poor and the elderly in an era of declining public support? If not, which groups are likely to suffer?

Can we protect the providers which serve the poor and elderly from reductions in public support for their services? Can we protect the education and research programs dependent on those services and their funding?

We found these questions difficult and troubling. We could not agree on answers, but perhaps our discussion will help move decision making in the right direction. If so, the Seventh Private Sector Conference will have served its purpose.

William G. Anlyan, M.D.

Acknowledgments

Without the support of the Duke Endowment, which has sponsored the Private Sector Conferences since their inception in 1977, this book would not have been possible.

William G. Anlyan

For Patricia Hodgson and Lynn Walker, who cheerfully performed the most tedious editorial and clerical chores, my special thanks.

Duncan Yaggy

Participants

John E. Affeldt, M.D., President, Joint Commission on the Accreditation of Hospitals

William G. Anlyan, M.D., Vice President for Health Affairs, Duke University

Karl Bays, Chairman of the Board and Chief Executive Officer, American Hospital Supply Corporation

John C. Beck, M.D., Professor of Medicine, University of California at Los Angeles

William Bevan, Ph.D., former Provost, Duke University (now Vice-President of the John D. and Catherine T. MacArthur Foundation)

Joseph A. Califano, Jr., Esq., Califano, Ross, and Heineman (former Secretary of Health, Education, and Welfare)

John W. Colloton, Director and Assistant to the President for Health Affairs, University of Iowa Hospitals and Clinics

John A. D. Cooper, M.D., President, Association of American Medical Colleges

Karen Davis, Ph.D., Professor, School of Hygiene and Health, Johns Hopkins University

Merlin K. DuVal, M.D., President, National Center for Medical Education

David M. Eddy, M.D., Director, Center for Health and Clinical Policy, Duke University

Paul Ellwood, Jr., M.D., President, InterStudy

E. Harvey Estes, Jr., M.D., Chairman, Department of Community and Family Medicine, Duke University Medical Center

Lynn Etheredge, Office of Management and Budget

Ashley H. Gale, Jr., The Duke Endowment

Eli Ginzberg, M.D., Director, Conservation of Human Resources, Columbia University

David A. Hamburg, M.D., John F. Kennedy School of Government, Harvard University

C. Rollins Hanlon, M.D., Director, American College of Surgeons

Joseph Lipscomb, Jr., Ph.D., Associate Professor of Public Policy Studies and of Community and Family Medicine, Duke University

Billy McCall, The Duke Endowment

J. Alexander McMahon, President, American Hospital Association

Donald MacNaughton, Hospital Corporation of America

Walter McNerney, J. K. Kellog Graduate School of Management (former President, Blue Cross Association, National Association of Blue Shield Plans)

Margaret Mahoney, President, The Commonwealth Fund

David Mechanic, Ph.D., Dean, Faculty of Arts and Sciences, Rutgers University

Alan Nelson, M.D., Trustee, American Medical Association

Tom E. Nesbitt, M.D., Urology Associates, Nashville, Tennessee

Joseph N. Onek, Esq., Onek, Klein, and Pharr

Uwe E. Reinhardt, Ph.D., Woodrow Wilson School of Public and International Affairs, Princeton University

Roscoe R. Robinson, M.D., Vice Chancellor for Medical Affairs, Vanderbilt University

David E. Rogers, M.D., President, The Robert Wood Johnson Foundation

Paul G. Rogers, Esq., Hogan and Hartson

James H. Sammons, M.D., Executive Vice President, American Medical Association

Charles A. Sanders, M.D., E. R. Squibb & Sons, Inc.

Jack K. Shelton, Manager, Employee Insurance Department, Ford Motor Company

Daniel C. Tosteson, M.D., Dean, Harvard Medical School

Richard S. Wilbur, M.D., Executive Vice President, Council of Medical Specialties

Session I

1. Providing Medical Care to the Elderly and Poor: A Serious Problem for the Downsizing 1980s

David E. Rogers

Providing responsibly and humanely for the elderly and indigent is going to be one of the most sensitive and difficult issues of this decade. A worsening national economic situation has led the public to place a much lower priority on providing health services, particularly tax-supported services, to our low-income citizens. Medicaid, neighborhood health centers, municipal hospitals, maternal and child health programs have fallen within the lengthening shadow of diminishing public concern.

Should these trends continue, we in the private sector may face very difficult circumstances in the years ahead. If we allow our immediate economic worries to dictate draconian reductions in support for the elderly and indigent, we may find America the scene of escalating confrontations between the haves and have-nots. On the other hand, if we are not responsive to the problems of our faltering economy we will end up in the same state.

Nowhere are these issues and trade-offs, or the need for thoughtful approaches, more apparent than in the arena of health care. Most Americans believe that health care should be available to all those who are sick or injured, regardless of economic or other circumstances. At the same time, most Americans also believe that there must be cuts in public spending for health care. Where to make the cuts without erasing the gains of the last several decades, or hurting the least fortunate among us, is the issue. It will take our best thinking to choose the right course.

There are many issues on which we could focus our discussion. But I believe that the major one is Medicaid: what should we do about our largest public sector health program for the poor? Given its size, all other issues are distinctly secondary. To set the stage, I propose to examine Medicaid with a high power lens. What has it accomplished? What are its problems? What might we suggest for dealing with them? I have discussed these issues with Dr. Robert Blendon and Thomas Maloney, colleagues with whom I have worked for nearly a decade, and their thoughts contributed importantly to the following analysis.

It has been almost seventeen years since President Lyndon Johnson flew to Independence, Missouri, to have former President Harry Truman join him in signing the legislation that created the Medicare and Medicaid programs. At the time the event was thought to mark an enduring American achievement.

But no one then realized that these programs would, by 1980, grow to pay for most of the health care received by 25 million elderly, 3.5 million disabled people, 10 million poor children, and 5 million unmarried, low-income parents —or that their care would cost the government more than $60 billion yearly.

Fifteen years later, faced with a worsening economy, upward pressures on public sector spending, and a powerful public mandate to reduce taxes and government expenditures, many of the nation's public and private sector leaders are now suggesting that we move away from these commitments of which we were so proud a decade ago.

This looming shift in our government's role reflects more than the wishes of a conservative administration in Washington. It mirrors a distinct and profound change in public attitudes toward domestic priorities. Prior to the election of the Reagan administration, the change was already being felt in state capitals across the country; Proposition 13 in California and Proposition 2½ in Massachusetts were only the most dramatic indications of growing public demands for governmental fiscal restraint and a sharp change in public opinion. In the early 1970s, national polls showed the public to be quite concerned about social issues including better health care, education, and welfare. Those polls also indicated a much higher level of confidence in the government's ability to manage these problems. But recent polls tell a different story. Social problems are not high on the public agenda; worries about the economy, inflation, and unemployment are way out ahead.

Add to this the anxieties created by events abroad, and the polls suggest the outlines of a growing consensus for a reordering of priorities, to place more emphasis on national security and less on human welfare. For the first time in many years, a majority (63 percent) of Americans believes that controlling inflation is worth a substantial cut in government spending, even in those programs they like best. In contrast, 27 percent oppose such cuts; 10 percent are unsure.

At the national level the Reagan administration set the goal of reducing public spending from a high of 23 percent of the Gross National Product (GNP) in 1981 to 19 percent beginning in 1984, a level last achieved at the end of the Eisenhower administration. (See figure 1.1.) Even so, defense expenditures are to increase sharply and significantly, which means that federal nondefense outlays will have to be reduced by $80 billion in 1983 and $104 billion in 1984. Health care outlays now constitute 13 percent of all nondefense spending. Clearly much of the savings must be taken there.

Similar decisions are being made at state levels. Education, public welfare, and health consume more than half of all state public expenditures, and they are major targets for reductions in future growth. Expenditures for health care programs are particularly vulnerable. They now account for one-third of state human welfare outlays. During the 1960s and 1970s, they grew 40 percent faster than any other human welfare expenditures.

The three largest public health care programs are Medicare, Medicaid, and a general category of health grants, which support maternal and child health,

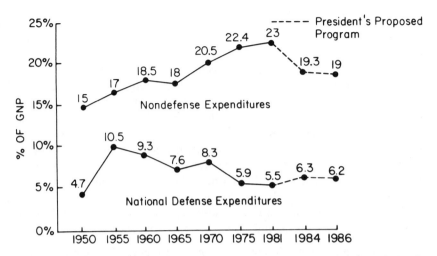

Figure 1.1. Federal spending as a share of the American economy, 1950–86

neighborhood health centers, family planning, and drug abuse and alcohol centers for the poor. These represent more than 75 percent of all public sector expenditures in health.

Within that grouping, certain health programs seem more likely than others to be curtailed. The most severe expenditure restrictions will probably be placed on those that primarily serve our poorer citizens: Medicaid and the special grant programs targeted on the health problems of our most disadvantaged. These programs are a prime target for two important reasons. First, the public does not wish to cut expenditures significantly for the elderly, which gives Medicare some protection. Second, there are widespread misunderstandings about the nature of Medicaid, who it serves and what it has done, and the public is less enamored with it. This makes it an even more appealing target.

What are the public's attitudes about public expenditures for health care for the poor? How is Medicaid perceived? Here the polls indicate ambivalence. On the one hand Americans say they are more concerned about the growth of medical care costs than about access to care or the quality of care. On the other, they continue to have a strong interest in obtaining better health care. Two-thirds of Americans say they are willing to spend even *more* public sector money than they do now to make sure better health care is available.

Why then the public doubts about Medicaid? They stem, I believe, from the tendency to define Medicaid as a welfare program; two-thirds of Americans are opposed to spending more on welfare programs. The term "human welfare" has sadly become a negative term. It used to mean "human well-being," but it now means "humans permanently on public relief." The most vulnerable public health care programs are those the general public views as "welfare programs masquerading as health care programs." This category includes neighborhood health centers and health care for pregnant women and poor children and youths, as well as Medicaid. These programs have become identified as another welfare payment to a group of undeserving ne'er-do-wells: unemployed adults and minorities.

How have these perceptions emerged? The answer is to be found on both sides of the political aisle. One side views Medicaid as another Great Society program that hasn't worked. These detractors contend that recipients are no healthier than they were before Medicaid and other governmentally financed health care programs. For them, dismantling these efforts is a socially responsible act. The other side continually stresses the inadequacies of these programs. They want more, not less, public spending for medical care. Foremost in their minds are the inequities and discontinuities that result from public health care coverage that is neither universal nor uniform.

Criticisms of these programs flow so thickly from both sides of the aisle that it is not surprising that the public believes that Medicaid is:

— A program to provide support primarily for potentially employable adults and minorities.
— Not successful in improving the health of recipients.
— Exceedingly, perhaps uncontrollably, inflationary due primarily to fraud, abuse, and misuse.
— Unimportant to the private health care institutions that provide care to employed Americans and their families.

A review of the facts suggests that none of these widely held beliefs is true. If we are to constructively downsize Medicaid expenditures, we need to be clear-eyed about them.

First, who actually receives help under the Medicaid program? A broad cross section of people benefit, primarily elderly people who are retired (38 percent), people who are blind or severely disabled (27 percent), and poor children (19 percent). Less than 30 percent of the program's funds pay for services for minorities.

The Medicaid program is in effect three distinct health care programs.

1. Elderly people who become poor in old age receive 38 percent of all expenditures. Most (75 percent) of these funds are used to provide nursing home care for people who, for most of their lives, were productive members of financially independent families. Most are now seventy, widowed, and unable to live alone. Fewer than 20 percent of these people are members of minorities.

2. The blind, mentally retarded, and physically disabled receive 27 percent of all expenditures. This program provides medical care (57 percent) and nursing home services (43 percent) for individuals with severe disabilities and higher than average needs for medical care.

3. Poor children and single-parent families, who compose almost two-thirds of those enrolled in the Medicaid program, receive a little more than one-third of all expenditures. This program provides primary medical care (99 percent) for a large number of children in poor single-parent families. Of expenditures

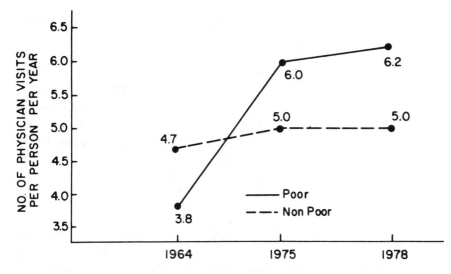

Figure 1.2. Per person physician visits for the poor and nonpoor, 1964–78

for this group, 55 percent are for children; 17 percent are for children below the age of six.

The percentage of total expenditures devoted to each of these categories varies greatly from state to state because the states have considerable latitude in choosing which programs to emphasize. How this will play out if the program is federalized remains to be seen.

Second, what of the belief that the Medicaid program has not done much to improve the health of its recipients? This charge is more difficult to answer. Medicaid and the other special health programs have dramatically improved the ability of poor people to enter the medical care system. Before their enactment, people with low incomes saw physicians far less often than middle class people; by the mid-1970s, this inequity was also eliminated, as figure 1.2 shows. Before Medicaid, poor elderly people received hospital care substantially less often than middle class elderly. As figure 1.3 demonstrates, this inequity had been erased by the mid-1970s. These are really monumental achievements, and I am surprised that we have not made more of them.

Can we prove that increased medical care makes poor people healthier? Obviously not, but it is a fact that the health of Americans, particularly the poor, began to improve when Medicaid, Medicare, and the other categorical health programs were enacted or expanded. These improvements, some of them dramatic, have continued ever since. No real increase in longevity was achieved for any age group between the mid-1950s and the advent of these public sector health programs. Then, beginning in 1968, life expectancy began to grow steadily for almost all age categories. Overall, age-adjusted death rates dropped by 21 percent over the period (figure 1.4). Infant death rates for blacks dropped a

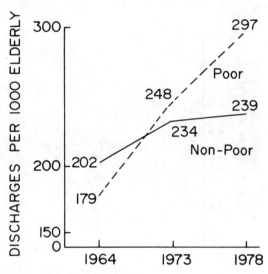

Figure 1.3. Hospital discharges for the poor and nonpoor elderly, 1964–78

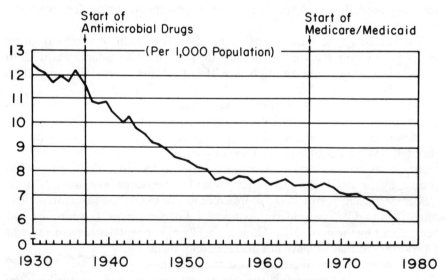

Figure 1.4. Age-adjusted death rates, United States, 1930–78

Source: Data from National Center for Health Statistics (slightly modified).

dramatic 45 percent (figure 1.5). This indicator is often used as a proxy measure for low income people because information on infant mortality by income groups is not recorded. Indeed there have been dramatic drops in eleven of fifteen major causes of American deaths. Perhaps more germane, there have also been significant decreases in the rates of death from diseases where medical

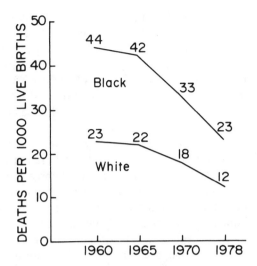

Figure 1.5. Infant mortality rates by race, 1960–78

care clearly can be lifesaving. These include influenza and pneumonia (40 percent), tuberculosis (70 percent), and diabetes (20 percent).

No set of public sector programs can claim direct credit for these impressive improvements. But they do coincide with the nation's most aggressive and successful effort to increase access to medical services for the poor and elderly.

Third, what of the costs—viewed by most as excessive, highly inflationary and markedly escalated by fraud and abuse? Actually, Medicaid costs per recipient are about the same as private medical costs for the general population. Here the evidence is solid. Contrary to popular belief, the average yearly medical expense for Medicaid recipients, despite probable increased burdens of illness, is only about 5 percent higher than the average private medical expense for a person of similar age in the population at large. That fraud or abuse exist in such a massive, complex program seems inevitable. But of what magnitude? Even if every claim of fraud, abuse, and overuse proved true, the net expense of any such failings is apparently not high enough to raise the costs per person of the program above the costs per capita of medical care for comparable, non-recipient Americans.

Why then have overall Medicaid costs increased 40 percent faster than total health expenditures over the past decade? The major reason is that the program has been successful in reaching people in need. Between 1968 and 1980 the number of poor people enrolled almost doubled, rising from eleven million to twenty-one million. In other words, in the main, total costs increased rapidly because each year many more people received care.

There is yet another reason for Medicaid's rising cost that logic demands we view positively. As the number of elderly has grown in our society, and deinstitutionalization programs have brought more mentally and physically disabled people into the community, both groups have become beneficiaries of the Medicaid program. Medicaid spending per elderly and disabled person is higher than average, primarily because these recipients so often are located in nursing homes. More than 75 percent of Medicaid expenditures for the elderly and more than 45 percent of those for the disabled go for nursing home care.

Fourth, what of the belief that Medicaid is not of much importance to the major private institutions that provide the bulk of care to Americans? Not so. Like it or not, the Medicaid program has become very important to the institutions that mainly serve people who are not Medicaid recipients. Medicaid now pays 11 percent of all hospital expenses across the country. More important, it represents a crucial source of reimbursement for care for some two hundred hospitals in the nation's largest cities. For example, in 1978, prior to the then impending cutbacks in Medicaid, these institutions already had reported deficits totaling more than $200 million. For many of these institutions Medicaid reimbursement has been critical to their continuing existence. For sixty-five of the nation's three hundred largest teaching hospitals, the need is even more compelling: Medicaid payments represent more than 25 percent of their total reimbursement. A few examples include the University of Pennsylvania Hospital in Philadelphia, the University of Chicago hospitals and clinics, University Hospital in Jackson, Mississippi, and the Children's Hospital of Los Angeles. These major teaching, research, and patient care centers provide services to thousands of people with private insurance. Further, they are the major source of highly specialized care for complex, difficult-to-treat illnesses. These institutions would be badly injured by severe cutbacks in Medicaid expenditures, particularly if they continue, as I believe they must, to treat the less fortunate.

There is yet another group of institutions that relies heavily on Medicaid. The majority of the nation's private nursing homes receive a substantial percentage of their revenues from the program. Medicaid now pays over 50 percent of all nursing home expenditures nationally. The future of these homes, which serve all income classes, would be seriously threatened by a significant withdrawal of Medicaid funds, and it might well cause immediate disruptions for thousands of private paying patients who use these homes.

Last, Medicaid reductions are to begin at a time when two groups of people who need Medicaid assistance will be increasing in numbers: the elderly and the recently unemployed. People in these groups who contributed to the program when they were employed taxpayers may now find their medical care seriously restricted precisely when they need help, unless we make the cutbacks with great care and precision.

Despite their shortcomings, Medicaid and associated public programs have played an important and generally beneficial role in our society. But the pressures to reduce public nondefense expenditures are now overwhelming, and it seems inevitable that these programs will bear the major brunt of the cutbacks.

The question is not "if," but "how" and "how much." It also bears emphasis that this will occur during a period when private giving and organized philanthropy can make up only a small part of the shortfall. When we compare the projected growth in private giving to health, education, welfare, environment, and the arts for the period 1982–84 with the increase required to offset federal budget cuts to those same areas, we find there is a modest discrepancy between the two! At the same time private foundations, although viewed with affection by universities, have comparatively little to contribute to fill that gap.

The dilemma facing public and private leaders is how to respond to the need to restrain the rapidly rising costs of these health care programs while continuing to provide the poor with vital medical services. Walking this tightrope will involve some uncomfortable trade-offs, particularly when it is more generally recognized that many of these publicly financed health care programs are not really more expensive per recipient than comparable medical care for the rest of us.

Where can the private sector play a role in all of this? The nation's leaders can choose from only two general strategies to accomplish their cost cutting. The first is administratively simple: substantially reduce the numbers of poor and nearly poor people who are covered by public sector health programs, and reduce the services provided to those deemed eligible. But this course may prove extraordinarily expensive over the long haul in both human and economic terms. No thoughtful person—in or out of government—wants to deny vital medical services to poor people who need them. No one, and least of all the physician, wants to return to the situation that existed in the pre-Medicaid era.

The private sector can and should help government take the second route, namely, to make highly selective, professionally determined cuts where they will do the least harm. This approach, while logical, will be vastly more difficult to implement. It will involve time, information, and the close collaboration of public officials, hospitals, physicians, dentists, nursing home directors, and community leaders. It will entail changes in how we currently pay for health care for the poor and the development of more conservative ways of organizing and providing that care.

Whether public officials will be willing to preserve the vital core of health programs for the poor by a precise and surgical approach to public expenditures remains uncertain. It will require a large investment of their time and energy. For them to feel this worthwhile may ultimately depend on the ability of private sector leadership to show which benefits of these health care programs are worth preserving.

Public awareness of the benefits the nation has derived from health care programs focused on our poor citizens may be the crucial factor in determining which tool—the meat ax or the scalpel— is chosen. Health professionals and public officials need first to increase the public understanding of these programs and of their merits. If public officials are to create the political consensus necessary to reduce public expenditures that minimize the sacrifices asked of those most in need, they must better understand where the programs have succeeded and where they have failed. I hope this conference will produce some practical ideas for opinion leaders in the health professions and government. I would also hope that we could agree that the route chosen should preserve the gains we have achieved in health care for the poor during the last decade and a half.

2. The Financial Support of Health Care for the Elderly and the Indigent: Economic Perspectives

Eli Ginzberg

This paper sets forth my understanding of the implications of the changing economic framework for the delivery of health care services to the elderly and the poor during the period 1982–90. Rather than use a conventional data-laden analysis, I thought it would be more useful if I presented my assessment of the certainties, probabilities, and possibilities that will determine the quantity and quality of health care likely to be available to the elderly and the poor in the 1980s.

Health Care System Cost

The federal government has reached a point in the evolution of its expenditure patterns where its share of the costs for Medicare and Medicaid approximates 10 percent of its total outlays. If not contained, health care expenditures will rise steeply in the years ahead. The pressure on the federal government is heightened when one recalls that so much of its budget is uncontrolled. To complicate matters further, Congress has eliminated the windfall resources that the government was able to obtain in years past as greater numbers of taxpayers were pushed into higher tax brackets by inflation. There is little or no prospect that the budget and appropriations committees of the Congress in the years ahead can ignore the expenditure increases implicit in current patterns of reimbursement.

The health care expenditures of many states have also escalated as a result of their role in the financing of Medicaid. In 1979 the combined state and local share of Medicaid expenditures amounted to about 4.6 percent of all state general expenditures, while absorbing 7.3 percent of all state revenues derived from state taxes and from local government transfers. This average obscures the current burden of Medicaid to those states with large indigent populations and reasonably liberal benefits, such as New York (14 percent), Massachusetts (12 percent), Rhode Island (11 percent), Connecticut (9 percent), and New Jersey (9 percent).[1] The governors successfully fought President Reagan's plan to place a cap on the annual outlays of the federal government for Medicaid, but in the process Congress reduced the amount of such federal expenditures over the next three years by a few percentage points, which (taking inflation into account) represents a marked reduction.

In the last few years more and more states have reduced the number of people eligible for Medicaid or restricted the range of services for which they are eligible. During the five months between December 1980 and May 1981, seventeen states adopted such restrictions, and as many more were considering similar limits.[2] In the absence of a marked improvement in their revenues, the states will be increasingly concerned with limiting their expenditures for Medicaid and other health care services for the elderly and the poor.

Even in the years when expenditures on behalf of the elderly and the poor grew rapidly, about 10 percent of the total population had shallow coverage.[3] Then too, most informed observers have found reason to question the *quality* of selected aspects of health care for the elderly and the poor, particularly nursing home services.[4] Without plan or intention, about 40 percent of all Medicaid funds went to the reimbursement of services for nursing home patients, but these funds were insufficient, even when supplemented by patient payments, to provide a satisfactory level of care for many who were institutionalized. These shortcomings, together with the other inequities and inadequacies of Medicaid coverage, explain the pressure for national health insurance and the reform of Medicaid during the 1970s. Neither movement succeeded in overcoming the political and economic barriers that blocked action.

Medicare has never covered as much as half of the health care expenditures for the elderly. Even with other public expenditures included (especially Medicaid payments for nursing home care), those sixty-five and over still had 37 percent of their health care costs paid by private sources.[5] This comparatively low coverage turned out to be less damaging than anticipated because of the sizable gains that Social Security recipients made in the 1970s as a result of higher benefit levels and overcorrections for inflation.[6]

There is broad agreement among health care analysts that one of the most dysfunctional consequences of Medicare and Medicaid has been the cost inflation resulting from the reimbursement practices adopted by Medicare. While the utilization estimates for Medicare and Medicaid proved reasonably accurate, expenditure outlays were greatly underestimated because cost reimbursement for hospitals and Medicare's usual, customary, and reasonable (UCR) reimbursement for physician fees pushed total outlays much higher than anticipated. One unsolved problem is the inflationary potential of the current system.

Five other factors may have a substantial impact on health care delivery for the elderly and the poor:

1. The numbers of older persons will rise steadily in the years ahead; growth will be most significant among those over seventy-five, the heaviest consumers of services.

2. No one knows how the economy will perform in the years ahead, but it is likely that unemployment will remain relatively high until the mid-1980s, if not longer. Considerable numbers of families may lose their health insurance as a result of unemployment.

3. The same trends are likely to increase the number of those eligible for

Medicaid and those who are close to the Medicaid cutoff point. This means that we must anticipate increases in the number of patients who will be unable to cover their health care bills, in whole or in part. In the Municipal Health Services Program, an ambulatory care demonstration in five large cities funded by the Robert Wood Johnson Foundation, there is scattered evidence that new patients are appearing at community health clinics in order to reduce their dollar outlays for health care.

4. Cost shifting is becoming more difficult. One goal of the Reagan Administration is to shift some of the cost for entitlement programs from the federal government to the private sector. Medicare has for some time paid less than its proportionate share of certain overhead items in its hospital reimbursement rates. Through legislation and administrative devices, the federal government, as well as some state governments, is increasing its efforts to shift greater responsibility onto private sector payers. However, the major source of flexibility is gone; hospital patients who are covered by commercial insurers are no longer fair game. Employers and trade unions are pressing their carriers to secure special discounts like those Blue Cross has been able to extract from many of its providers.[7] The potential for cost shifting is narrowing all the time.

5. Medical schools located in or close to urban concentrations of the poor must now anticipate that more patients of limited means will seek care at their hospitals. Faced with level or declining revenues for research and development, and for educational and teaching activities, many urban health science centers will find it difficult to meet increasing demands for services from the indigent. A major health science center in New York is considering when it must return to a practice of yesteryear and send nonpaying patients to a neighboring municipal hospital.

In sum, there is considerable noise in the system. Health care services to the elderly and the poor are being compromised by the unsolved problems of the post Medicare and Medicaid period; the tightening budgetary position of the federal and state governments; the uncontrolled inflationary influences in the health care system; and the worsening economic outlook.

Efforts Constraining Costs

Federal government. The federal government has initiated a number of efforts to slow the increase in its expenditures for the elderly and the poor, including:

— Tightening limits on outlays for Medicare and Medicaid.
— Instructing the Secretary of the Department of Health and Human Services (HHS) to propose plans for prospective reimbursement.
— Attempting to cap outlays for Medicare and Medicaid by limiting increases to an inflationary index.
— Experimenting with efforts to offer Medicare recipients the alternative of Health Maintenance Organization (HMO) coverage.

— Planning to shift coverage for employed persons over sixty-five to their employers' health benefit plan.
— Designating Medigap and other private insurance benefits as the primary sources of health care reimbursement for elderly patients, with Medicare serving as a secondary reimbursement source.
— Allowing states to become prudent purchasers for their Medicaid populations.
— Eliminating extras in reimbursements to hospitals for Medicare patients.
— Reducing support for federally supported community health care centers and other health programs.
— Increasing copayments by beneficiaries for Supplemental Insurance benefits.
— Requiring small copayments by Medicaid patients at point of use.

State government. At the state level, one can identify the following responses to the dollar crunch:

— Cutbacks in eligibility and in coverage for Medicaid.
— Intensified efforts to control the expansion of nursing home capacity in order to limit the state's commitment to pay for an increased number of patients.
— Growing recourse to state authority to regulate hospital care reimbursements for Medicaid and Blue Cross patients.
— Further efforts to transfer patients in state institutions to programs and facilities to which the federal government contributes.
— Modest experimentation with new approaches, such as home care, for selected groups of patients who might otherwise require institutionalization.

County and local government. Steps at the local level have included:

— Sales, leases, and management contracts under which local governments turn over control of their hospitals to for-profit or nonprofit hospital chains, in the hope and expectation of limiting prospective liabilities of tax payers for health care expenditures.
— Closed-end allocations to medical facilities in order to contain future costs.
— Efforts to reduce, merge, or close down health facilities and programs that no longer provide essential services to the poor.

Private sector. The pressure on voluntary hospitals and physicians shows itself in these ways:

— Hospitals with inadequate cash flow, limited philanthropic support, and locations in deteriorating neighborhoods are deciding to merge or close, a trend that is likely to accelerate in the years ahead as the competition for insured patients worsens. (Many of these hospitals have cared for signi-

ficant numbers of the poor and near poor, both as inpatients and out-patients.)
— In response to governmental cutbacks for Medicaid, financially marginal voluntary hospitals have been transferring patients whose entitlements are exhausted to public institutions. (In a period of six months, Cook County Hospital experienced a fourfold increase in such transfers, some of which involved patients whose lives were endangered as a result.)
— An increasing number of voluntary hospitals are seeking links with existing community health centers in the hope of increasing their flow of in-patients and thereby enlarging their revenue base.
— Other voluntary hospitals are looking for opportunities to tie into their operations organized and/or unorganized physicians who practice in lower income areas for the purpose of assuring themselves a larger and more reliable flow of patients, a high proportion of whom are covered by Medicaid or private insurance.
— Experiments under way in both New Jersey and Maryland aim to "socialize" the costs of unpaid hospital bills by distributing them among all third-party payers.
— In a few locations, state government and Blue Cross have made funds available to assist voluntary institutions that provide a high volume of ambulatory care to nonpaying patients.
— Scattered evidence that physicians who are encountering difficulty in developing a practice are beginning to make house calls. (If the trend accelerates, it should enable some of the elderly to avoid institutionalization).
— Scattered evidence that physicians are beginning to compete on price to attract and hold larger numbers of elderly and poor patients.
— Emergi-centers and other for-profit innovations designed to deliver ambulatory care at a relatively low cost are developing.

In sum, the early responses point to:

— Reductions in facilities and programs serving elderly and poor patients.
— An effort at all levels of government to contain health care outlays, which will have an adverse effect on access for the elderly and poor.
— The limited capacity of the private sector to compensate for reductions in governmental funding.
— Increased competition for patients through new delivery modes and lower prices that may moderate to some extent the reduction in access now in prospect.

Radical Proposals

The fiscal pressures on federal, state, and local governments may be so great that the modest adjustments identified above may not provide as much relief as legislators will consider necessary or desirable. Further complications may arise in the private sector as a result of accelerated mergers and closures of hospitals that will leave many elderly and poor groups without reasonable access. Further, many voluntary hospitals may find themselves in such weakened financial condition that they will be forced to cut back, or eliminate completely, services to patients who are not insured. As a result, more radical proposals are now under discussion. They include proposals aimed at providing a voucher alternative for Medicare and Medicaid recipients that would enable them to seek coverage from an HMO. It is assumed that this would be less costly and/or more comprehensive and better suited to their needs. An analysis of the Medicaid voucher by Frank Sloan suggests that it will be cost increasing, not cost reducing.[8]

In the case of Medicare vouchers, several factors must be clarified, including the right of those who select vouchers to shift back to the present system, the degrees of freedom allowed HMOs to select among Medicare patients, the value of the voucher, and so forth. Some of the best informed students of HMOs do not expect them to enroll more than 10 or 12 percent of the population by 1990.[9] Hence, it is unlikely that the voucher-HMO route will absorb more than a small proportion of all elderly and poor. Moreover, in the absence of much broader and deeper demonstrations than have yet been undertaken, it would be highly venturesome to postulate that the voucher-HMO approach would result in lower total outlays than the extant system. In theory, they might; in practice, the odds appear to be the other way.[10]

Procompetition bills now in the federal hopper seek to reduce the tax expenditure costs involved in the present system of employer-employee purchase of group health insurance. It is unlikely that Congress will place a ceiling on these expenditures that would force current beneficiaries to pay taxes on benefits above the cap. However, it is conceivable a sufficiently high ceiling will be established so that health benefits now tax free to the employer or the employee will someday be capped. The tax savings to the federal government from such an action would be modest until the second half of the decade, but thereafter they could be of growing importance. The Congressional Budget Office has estimated the losses from employer contributions for medical benefit plans to be $16.6 billion in 1982.[11] My guess is that Congress will not place a cap on tax-free health care benefits, except as part of a comprehensive tax reform package that will deprive the upper income groups of comparable tax benefits.

Since most of the procompetition health bills include provisions to cover the entire population and to protect all individuals and families from catastrophic costs, they carry with them additional outlays. Alain Enthoven estimated in 1980 that his Consumer Choice Health Plan carried an extra price tag of $22.4 billion in 1978 dollars.[12] In my view there is little or no prospect that Congress will pass new health legislation that carries an additional significant up-front cost, no matter what the sponsors promise about long-term economies. There are rumors afloat that some congressional staffers are exploring the transformation of Medicare from an entitlement to a means-tested program. In light of the quick retreat of the administration on the Social Security front, with respect to both reducing payments to early retirees and eliminating the minimum benefit, it is hard to conceive that a means-tested Medicare is a likely development in the near or midterm. I would rule this out for the indefinite future.

The most radical procompetition bill (HR850—the National Health Care Reform Act of 1981) would let the market decide what insurance carriers can profitably sell. Government would play at most a minor role in stipulating the nature of the coverage. I believe that most hospitals, insurance carriers, and medical leaders are fundamentally opposed to such a radical shift in medical insurance. Moreover, I have little faith that a free market would result in lower total expenditures. And I am reasonably certain that the elderly and poor would be further disadvantaged if it were enacted.

In sum, I do not expect any of these radical proposals to be enacted in the next few years. An increase in health care expenditures from the present level of 9.4 percent of GNP to 11 or 12 percent would have to occur before any would be seriously considered.

Impact and Implications

The United States is in a period of stress and strain as regards the financing of health care, especially for the elderly and poor, and my expectations are shaped accordingly:

Short term (1982–85). Some parts of the gains in utilization registered by the poor since 1965 will be lost as Medicaid coverage is cut back and the private sector finds itself less able to provide free care and care below cost. Continuing high unemployment will increase the numbers of persons with no coverage or inadequate coverage. The number of hospitals and nursing homes available to the elderly and poor is likely to be reduced in response to the unfavorable financial environment. There will be some compensation for these adverse trends in a shift from inpatient to ambulatory care, which will make it possible to stretch the available dollars. The substantial increase in the number of physicians per capita will contribute to such a shift.

The several efforts of government and other third-party payers to increase copayments by users will lower the demand for health care services by the elderly and poor.

The effort to shift costs from the public to the private sector will continue, but the scale of such transfers will be limited by the constraints under which most providers in the private sector will be operating.

The steady deterioration of most health science centers in urban areas carries a further threat to the elderly and poor, who have been accustomed to receiving considerable free care or care below cost from these providers.

As providers of last resort, municipal institutions are likely to be under increasing pressure to provide services for larger numbers of the elderly and poor at a time when their budgets will be severely constrained. They will be forced to ration the services they provide. The odds are that they will try to give some care to all who seek it and that they will be forced to restrict the numbers who receive adequate treatment.

If the federal government cuts back radically on its funding of rural and urban health care centers, as is likely, there is a danger that particular population groups, such as low income minorities in rural areas, who had limited access to care prior to 1965, will again face serious access problems.

Middle term (1986–90). The pressures on the federal and state governments to contain their total expenditures, including their health care expenditures, will be significantly affected by the trends in the U.S. economy during the next eight years. If inflation and unemployment remain relatively high and economic growth remains relatively low, the pressures on government to hold down expenditures will be very great. But if the economy does reasonably well, the budgetary situation will be less likely to force a radical retrenchment in health care.

As I have argued elsewhere, we will not be able to avoid reassessing our Social Security System, but it is now unclear whether OASDI or OASDI+HI will be the focus of such a reassessment.[13] It would make considerable sense to look at the combined needs of the elderly for income and health benefits to see whether some significant improvement could be obtained by a comprehensive rather than a piecemeal approach to restructuring. But the difficulties inherent in such a broad reassessment should not be minimized.

I would expect that Medicare will not remain intact through the 1980s, although the lines that a restructuring effort is likely to take are not clear to me. Significant dollar savings could result only from a reduction in days of hospitalization and a ceiling on nursing home care. But demographic trends, family structure, and the economic outlook are unfavorable. It may be necessary for the United States to begin a discussion of constraints on expensive medical interventions for old people who are approaching the ends of their lives.

There are likely to be substantial changes in the delivery system in the decade ahead resulting from the reduction of hospitals and hospital beds, the growth of HMOs, the increase in physicians, the larger role of for-profit enterprises, and so forth. Surely some of these should contribute to cost and price containment; to the extent that they do, they should ease somewhat the unfavorable outlook for health care services for the elderly and poor.

In the event that the economy goes into a serious tailspin and fails to extricate itself quickly, one must allow for the possibility that the financial underpinnings of insurance coverage for the public, hospital revenues, and physicians' earnings could be so seriously jeopardized that a renewed effort for a radical transformation of the system based on national health insurance would succeed. I do not expect this to happen but such a possibility cannot be ruled out.

Conclusion: Ten Lessons from Recent Experience

Congress did not appreciate the financial commitments involved in the enactment of Medicare and Medicaid. Because of favorable economic and revenue conditions, these large, expensive entitlement programs were able to become firmly rooted. In the process they contributed to structural changes in the rest of the health care system that triggered a steep acceleration of costs. For a decade Congress and to a lesser extent the states have tried to gain some control over the system, with only modest success.

In the budget resolution of 1981 the Reagan administration tried to cap and reduce the rate of increase in its outlays for Medicaid through prospective budgeting. Whether and how well prospective budgeting will work remains to be seen, but it should provide some relief to governments faced with the need to rein in their expenditures.

At the same time the "market" is working in some (even many) respects— with hospitals increasingly under pressure, the physician supply expanding rapidly, competition for patients intensifying, HMOs experiencing a continuing growth, a shift from inpatient to outpatient settings proceeding apace, and for-profit enterprises becoming ever more conspicuous in the delivery of services. These market forces will likely turn out to be of greater and more lasting significance in the restructuring of our health care system than financial reforms sought by governments.

However, it is hard to see how the decade of the 1980s will result in any significant gains in health care for the elderly and poor. My hope is that their care will not seriously erode. Both government and the private sector are obliged to see that it does not. They are more likely to succeed if they attend to the lessons of our recent experience.

Lesson 1. It is a dangerous mistake to rush the passage of major pieces of legislation. Medicaid was never really discussed by anybody in Congress; instead, it was the result of a deal which brought it in on the tail of Medicare. By circumventing the usual legislative process we didn't get a chance to access public opinion or to discover the hidden problems. We failed to understand some important consequences of the Medicaid legislation, one of which was the unexpected development that a very large part of Medicaid would go for the maintenance of old people in nursing homes.

Lesson 2. In our federal/state relationship, it is impossible to deliver anything like a uniform level of service, no matter how the federal and state governments work together, because we start from such different places. Under Medicaid, the federal government contributes as much as 83 percent of the cost for the poorest states, in an effort to compensate for their poverty. Yet there is unequivocal evidence that this is not the way it works because the poor states, or the states that are indifferent, just won't come up with their part of the money, even to take advantage of federal matching at very advantageous rates.

This is a particularly important lesson to bear in mind with all the discussion about federalization. Federalization would probably mean that a large number of the more liberal states, or the richer states, would simply not receive from the federal government funding commensurate with the level of services they give.

Lesson 3. There is nothing earth shattering about increasing health care expenditures from 6 percent to 9 percent of the GNP. I think we can even go from 9.5 to 12, 13, or 14 percent without breaking the country over the next years. But, at some point, there needs to be closure in our system of financing.

Lesson 4. We are in real difficulty with respect to the aged because the services to them are confounding and compounding all the time. They need some health care. A lot of them need maintenance care, a place to live, and somebody to help them take care of themselves. And, very important, people all continue to die. Over 30 percent of Medicare expenditures are for patients who are dead within twelve months. That does not mean that they should not have been in a hospital. It does not mean that they should not have had care. But in a time of increasingly limited resources some considerable part of that care is questionable because it is dying care for patients with no real prospects of improving.

Lesson 5. We must relate open-ended entitlements to the power of providers in our system. In 1964, New York City spent from all sources about $3 billion for health care and in 1978, $10 billion. In that same period of time, the population of New York City declined by about half a million people. I do not think there was any significant improvement in the quantity or the quality of the health care that the poor got. So, something else changed: a tremendous increase in discharges per thousand of the elderly from hospitals, as can be seen in Dr. Rogers' figure 1.5.

Providers are in a very powerful position to use patients with entitlements to meet all kinds of needs—good, bad, and indifferent—and that is what has happened. Neither Reagan, nor the Democrats, nor the Republicans, nor anyone else can operate very long with open-ended budgets. Some kind of prospective budgeting or capping of entitlements is essential. There is no way of maintaining the practices of the recent past.

Lesson 6. We must try to distinguish between those high cost patients who ought to be high cost because they can be returned to functionality and those high cost patients who ought to be in a caring system with pain control because they are dying. Dying care consumes a significant part of Medicare money because, as one of the consequences of Western medical progress, we have lost all perception of the nature of death in our society. We seem unwilling to accept the fact that people are going to die.

I'd like to tell you about a favorite cousin who should not have had any medical intervention yet whose dying costs were $60,000. She was severely ill, suffering from emphysema. She was admitted to a major academic health center where she underwent cardiac catheterization. Following the catheterization she had a quadruple bypass, and was then in a coma for thirty days before she died. Unless the people who control the medical care system exercise some discipline, the system can run away with itself.

Lesson 7. I strongly believe that local planning is essential. Bureaucrats in Washington, D.C., cannot be expected to figure out the level and quality of care in relationship to local resources. Those estimates must be made locally in order to coordinate available resources with needs. Each provider wants to go his own way, but neither the state, the city, nor anyone else is going to let that happen.

Lesson 8. It is important to watch the relationship between the number of physicians and the cost of the system. We are now on the brink of a tremendous increase in the supply of physicians. No matter what is done to hospital capacity, no matter how much more sensible physician intervention becomes, physicians who have spent a long time getting trained will want to use their skills to make a living.

Lesson 9. The question is not whether government will decrease its health care expenditures, but how it will decrease them. There are good and bad ways of doing it, and that should be the issue before this group. First of all, it is very important to see that actions are taken on every level—local, federal and state— to make sure that people who must get medical care are not rejected. One of the jobs of the private sector is to make sure the government does not walk away from its legitimate obligations to meet the health needs of the poor. Further, we need to socialize the cost of unpaid medical bills. Otherwise, certain hospitals will be jeopardized, further reducing the access of the poor to the facilities that they need. It is the hospitals that are providing the extra services where the poor are that will go under first.

Lesson 10. We must pay attention to excessively high cost facilities because of their capacity to increase the cost of the system. Why, for instance, does Chicago need six medical schools? Excess capacity tends to draw dollars in and give very little return to the public.

Notes

1. U.S. Bureau of the Census, *Statistical Abstract of the United States: 1980*, 101st ed. (Washington, D.C.: 1980); U.S. Department of Health and Human Services, *Expenditures for Public Assistance Programs, Fiscal Year 1979* (Washington, D.C.: Office of Research and Statistics, SSA, 1980), table 4.24, p. 170.

2. The Intergovernmental Health Policy Project, *Recent and Proposed Changes in State Medicaid Programs: A Fifty State Survey* (Washington, D.C.: October 1981).

3. Congressional Budget Office, *Profile of Health Care Coverage: The Haves and the Have Nots* (Washington, D.C.: March 1979).

4. B. Vladeck, *Unloving Care: The Nursing Home Tragedy* (New York: Basic Books, 1980).

5. C. R. Fisher, "Difference by Age Groups in Health Care Spending," *Health Care Financing Review* 1 (1980): 89.

6. E. Ginzberg, "The Social Security System," *Scientific American* 246 (1982): 51–57.

7. E. Ginzberg et al., "The Expanding Physician Supply and Health Policy: The Clouded Outlook," *Milbank Memorial Fund Quarterly* 59 (1981): 508–41.

8. F. Sloan, "Medicaid Vouchers: Prospects and Problems," paper prepared for the 1981 Commonwealth Fund Forum, Medical Care for the Poor: What Can States Do in the 1980s?, Philadelphia, August 9–12, 1981.

9. L. D. Brown, personal communication.

10. Blue Cross and Blue Shield Associations, *Competition and Consumer Choice: A Third Party Payer's Perspective— Medicare Vouchers* (Washington, D.C.: September 1981).

11. Congressional Budget Office, *Tax Expenditures: Current Issues and Five Year Budget Projections for Fiscal Years 1982–1986* (Washington, D.C.: September 1981), p. 27.

12. A. C. Enthoven, *Health Plan: The Only Practical Solution to the Soaring Cost of Medical Care* (Reading, Mass.: Addison-Wesley, 1980).

13. Ginzberg, "The Social Security System," pp. 51–57.

3. Response

Uwe E. Reinhardt

I found these two papers very illuminating, and the forecasts within them very disturbing. Some of the numbers in Dr. Rogers' paper are new to me. For instance, the numbers comparing health care expenditures for Americans in general with expenditures for Medicaid beneficiaries are interesting and important. The central theme of his paper, I think, is that we should take pride in the achievements of Medicare and Medicaid over the last two decades.

During the 1980 election campaign, some politicians argued that Americans are worse off now than they were in 1960. If, however, we look at GNP per capita, at its distribution, at health status, access to health care, civil rights, and many other measures, we must conclude that we are infinitely better off than we were in 1960. As Dr. Rogers said, we should take pride in what has been achieved. The Great Society was not a failure, nor was Medicaid. We still have gaps, but these gaps do not negate the gains that have been made. I am glad that an observer of Dr. Rogers' stature said this, and I promise to quote him widely on this point henceforth.

Dr. Ginzberg's approach is to survey the world, write down what he sees, and then ask what all this means. Just in case you are stymied, he then proceeds to lay it out for you.

One cannot disagree with Dr. Ginzberg's perceptions. He perceives a growing need for health care for the aged and for the poor. He perceives an unwillingness or an inability to meet that need with the application of public funds. And he has some thoughts about what we should do in the short run and in the long run. I want to comment on his long-run solutions. Specifically, before we cave in and adapt our policy prescriptions to the perceived constraints, let us examine once more the extent to which these constraints are beyond our control.

I first want to call your attention to the manner in which we discuss social problems in America. We do talk in terms of constraints and trade-offs that are seen as exogenous and beyond our control. We treat this whole dilemma in which we find ourselves as something God imposed upon us poor Americans, as something we must endure because we do not have the necessary resources to escape these dire trade-offs. I think that is a cheap trick! Our problem is as much a reflection of our moral standards—or, really, lack of them—as it is the manifestation of externally imposed economic or technical constraints. America today is wealthier than it has ever been before. Says who that we cannot meet the needs of our poor and our aged? No, the real problem in America is that we are beset, and increasingly governed, by a bunch of narcissistic, pampered youngsters who have no couth. That is the central theme of anything I would write on this topic.

At any point in time in society there are those too young to work, those too old to work, and those who work. There is nothing we can do about the age distribution now. But the categorization of those too young to work and those too old to work is in part a social choice. We have increasingly allowed the young not to work and forbidden the old to work even if they would like to work. The dependency ratio is, thus, a function of retirement age. If we postpone retirement age to seventy, then the dependency ratio is about 30 percent: for every person retired there will be two working. If, on the other hand, we keep the present retirement pattern, the dependency will be 50 percent, which means that for every person retired there is one working. Clearly there is some choice. We must look seriously at this question of retirement age. When people are as vigorous as people now are when they get to sixty-five, it is silly to retire them at that age. The first constraint then is movable.

Let us next turn to the plight (so-called) of those who are gainfully employed in the marketplace. They are given to the lament that they have to share with others the pie they bake. Remarkably, they seem to take it as given that they have legal and moral title to the entire pie. Our politicians egg them on in this belief, and so do sundry other social commentators who ought to know better.

Not too long ago I heard a business school professor lament that his students faced a marginal tax rate of 40 percent so soon after receiving their MBA degrees. He expected us to flood the floor with tears of compassion for these youngsters. Most of the businessmen in the audience did, indeed, mellow with empathy. Should they have? I would argue that we have here a breakdown of pedagogy. My point is this: have these pitiable, freshly baked MBAs and their bleeding-heart mentors ever wondered who financed a good portion of the human capital these youngsters own after graduating with an MBA?

By "human capital" I mean the education and training society gave these youngsters. Most of what they earn upon graduation is, in fact, a financial return on that human capital, rather than a return on the brawn and muscle with which they entered the world. Although an MBA graduate can be said to have contributed something to the financing of his or her human capital in the form of foregone wages, the bulk of that capital has been financed by parents, alumni, and/or anonymous taxpayers, many of whom may be retired when the MBA finally starts to work (after close to a quarter century's period of eating and taking, taking, taking).

In principle, those who financed the MBA's human capital should get a return on that financing. The taxes our poor MBAs pay can be viewed as part of that repayment. And because these MBAs do not seem possessed of either the intellect or the couth to grasp this fact, perhaps the time is at hand to teach them manners in a more forceful way. Specifically, I propose that all college students should be made to *borrow* and cover out of their own future earnings the entire full cost of their undergraduate and graduate education. In other words, I would like to see us stop giving handouts to youngsters who have no moral claim on these handouts and divert the resources so garnered to the poor and aged who often have few options left.

Table 3.1. Government expenditures as a percentage of gross national product (United States)

Year	Federal	State and Local	Total
1970	20.6%	11.0%	31.6%
1975	23.0	11.5	34.5
1979	21.1	10.1	31.2
1980	22.9	10.2	33.1

Note: Includes government expenditures on goods and services, transfer payments, and trust account transactions with the public (e.g., Social Security payments and unemployment compensation).
Source: Tax Foundation, Inc., *Facts and Figures on Government Finance*, 1981, table 23, p. 36.

What this would mean in practice is the cessation of all state, federal, and local institutional subsidies to higher education. Students would then have to borrow for their education, maybe even from pension funds. These loans should be made available, but not subsidized. Loans should be made on the same terms as any business loans and with the same risks. Students would have to repay the loans entirely, with interest, over their working lives. We might then be able to lower their Social Security taxes, and their bellyaching would stop.

Associated with a human being is a life cycle cash flow. In the early years and in the later years, the cash outflow is larger than the inflow; in the intervening years, the cash inflow exceeds what one actually should need for consumption. We must teach our narcissistic youngsters to manage this life-cycle cash flow prudently.

In Europe they have been talking about a third leg of social insurance. They have health insurance, they have regular pensions, and they are now talking about insurance for long-term medical and social care. A law mandating long-term care insurance would require working people to put aside a large amount of money to pay for nursing home care when they are old, to prevent their becoming wards of the state.

Some people never have a cash inflow large enough to make their life cycle cash flow balance over their lifetimes. Can we ignore them or will we have compassion for them? The political philosophy in vogue now seems to reflect a total absence of compassion. I consider that a real outrage. Once again, the main economic problem we have in America is a lack of compassion for these people, and not a lack of resources.

We have been told that the government has gobbled up an ever larger share of the GNP. See table 3.1 for the percentages between 1970 and 1980 of federal, state, and local shares, and the total as percentages of the GNP. When I put these tables together, I had anticipated being able to show that our government is, indeed, eating up an ever bigger share of our GNP. When I looked at the numbers, however, I found that such was not the case. Thirty-one percent in 1970, thirty-one percent in 1979; state and local governments' take, as a percentage of GNP, has not increased at all.

Table 3.2 compares the growth of the public sector in other nations with our

Table 3.2. Government expenditures as a percentage of gross domestic product (selected countries)

Country	1978	1980	Increase
Canada	36.0	40.1	11.4%
France	38.5	46.3	20.3
West Germany	40.5	46.1	13.8
Japan	25.4	31.6	24.4
Netherlands	48.1	60.4	25.6
Sweden	46.1	63.2	37.1
United Kingdom	41.1	44.3	7.8
United States	32.0	33.1	3.4

Source: Fifty-first Annual Report, Bank for International Settlements, June 1981, p. 24.

growth over the last decade. Two things stand out. One, we have the smallest public sector in the world with the exception of Japan. Second, our public sector grew only three percent over the entire decade. In all other nations the growth was much, much higher.

We make much of the fact that we are a "pluralistic, heterogeneous" society. What a godsend that is! It gives us a perfect excuse for the considerable social pathos at the fringe of our society. We use that excuse all the time. "Don't blame us for the pathos," we say, "Blame God, for making us so heterogeneous." Although heterogeneity may add to the problem of coping with social pathos, there must surely be a limit to the number of debits we can ethically debit to that account. The fact is that we don't spend a lot on social pathos, the Reverend David Stockman's mutterings to the contrary notwithstanding. Indeed, I put to you the proposition that there is less social pathos in Europe and in neighboring Canada mainly because they are not as afraid as we are to apply resources to its elimination.

Over forty years ago Chief Justice Hughes said: "The security of the republic will be found in the treatment of the poor and the ignorant. In our indifference to their misery and helplessness lies disaster." I could not think of a more appropriate citation on which to end my commentary.

4. Response

Karl Bays

So many politicians, bureaucrats, reporters, people of all kinds bemoan the total cost of health care. Nine and a half percent of the GNP is somehow viewed as being a very, very high percentage to be paying for health care. Donald MacNaughton said recently that no one really knows how high or low that number should be, and I agree with him. It seems to me that this group should try to analyze the total expenditure. Most people feel that we invest enough in health care in total, but many perceive it to be poorly administered or badly distributed. Public awareness is very important in setting the agenda for the future. This issue should be discussed as we talk over the next couple of days.

Discussion

Mr. J. Alexander McMahon: There does not appear to be a vast difference between the cost of services for the indigent and the cost of services for the population as a whole. The government complains about the rate of increase in appropriations for Medicaid. In order to avoid a simplistic solution, Dr. Rogers suggests, "We must make highly selective, professionally determined cuts where they will do the least harm." My question is: why do we not take a look at how we might make highly selective, professionally determined cuts in the delivery of health services to all people, indigent and otherwise?

Dr. David Rogers: I thoroughly agree. I see a fair amount of evidence that business, insurers, the hospital industry, labor, and all kinds of coalitions are beginning to look at that.

Dr. Merlin K. DuVal: Dr. Ginzberg talked about the proportion of Medicare dollars that is spent in the last year of life. I would ask whether this isn't precisely what the program was put in place to take care of?

Having made that observation, I am forced to ask myself about Dr. Ginzberg's other question: when are we going to bring professional disciplines into the decision-making process about who is to live and who is to die? I would ask: what other groups in society might you turn to to make that kind of decision?

Dr. Eli Ginzberg: From my limited exposure and experience I suspect that too much health care money is being spent on many of those dying people, particularly people with no families who become the object of research and training experience in the medical schools. Medical students have to learn. They also represent an earning asset to an institution. I would simply say that there needs to be more review of the 30 percent of Medicare dollars that is being spent on dying people. I attach no importance to that figure except to say that it is big enough to look at and to compel us to distinguish between people who ought to be treated at high expense and people who should not be treated at high expense.

Further, a profession may not be able to come up with society's answers alone, but it surely has a responsibility to lead the discussion. I do not believe that physicians in our society can determine who is going to live and who is going to die. But I believe they do have to begin to talk about these issues. And it seems that, where families are active and where they are dealing with long-term physicians, there is more control over dying than there is when people are isolated and without protection.

Dr. John C. Beck: I would like to ask about terminal illness. If it is a problem, how are we going to deal with it?

There is another side to this issue. When we look at the elderly and their treatment in our acute tertiary care institutions, we find around four remediable problems that are missed at the time of each elderly person's discharge. Those remediable problems are often the kind that make the difference between the elderly person remaining functionally independent in the community or going to an institution, be it a nursing home or a board and care institution.

Two other questions: One, I want to know what birth rate assumptions Dr. Reinhardt used when he calculated the dependency ratio. Two, would Dr. Rogers explain how a "highly selective" trimming of health care expenditures would be made, since that becomes an institutional problem in the final analysis?

Professor Uwe E. Reinhardt: The data were taken from *Toward a National Retirement Income Policy*, from the president's Commission on Pension Policy.

Dr. David Rogers: One of the points I was trying to make—and this was a piece of data that surprised me—is the realization that it does not really cost much more to take care of people under Medicaid. That makes me suspect that it is going to be quite difficult to trim it enormously, although I am sure a great deal of money is expended that does not go directly to care services.

I have two comments I want to address to Dr. Ginzberg. First, I'm a little worried about the corner you are painting yourself into with that 30 percent figure for Medicare costs for people in their last year of life. If we knew which 30 percent were going to die, we might design care rather differently. As a physician, however, I'm not willing to play Russian roulette. Second, I will agree that we ought to collect those data, but I will bet the anecdote you related about your cousin is the striking exception rather than the rule. I don't see that happen very often. We let lots of people die who should die. The aberrant situation you describe happens in perhaps 3 percent of cases.

Dr. Ginzberg: The whole question of continuous decision making in complicated, chronic situations of the aged is a real challenge. I obviously do not expect you as a physician to deny treatment to an older person in a reversible situation. But when you reach the point of knowing that it is not reversible anymore, you should stop aggressive treatment and take some alternative measures.

I did not consider it a compliment to American medicine when a physician friend of mine sent a colleague of his from Europe back to a European hospice when he was diagnosed as having irreversible cancer. He had much more humane, much more useful, and much less expensive treatment there than he could have found here. I think our system is out of control. The dollars are inviting what I would call heroic interventions to go on way beyond the time they ought to.

Dr. James H. Sammons: It seems to me that we are mixing apples and oranges. First of all, let me tell you that we agree completely with the need for reevaluation of the problem. As a matter of fact, the AMA Board of Trustees just recently approved a proposal that we hope will stimulate the development of a rational, reasonable, and attainable national health policy, developed for and by the private sector. Since the first day that HEW was in existence it has not been able to do that. Government seems incapable of doing it. Maybe the private sector will have more luck. Whether it does or not, at least the AMA is going to give it a try.

Having said that and recognizing that we share the belief that the whole system needs another look, it seems to me that we continuously fall into the trap of discussing Medicaid as though the numbers were accurate. I do not think the numbers are accurate at all. We talk about the health care delivery system for the poor and we aggregate it with a tremendous amount of nonhealth care and custodial care, where attending physicians are not needed. If it were not for regulations that cause physicians to visit nursing homes at periodic intervals, costs would be lower.

The Medicaid legislation mixes up health care with entitlements, with custodial treatment, and with benefits for total disabilities that are not being pursued medically. These figures do not reflect what it costs to take care of the poor. If you believe the statistics that come out of HHS, and I see no reason not to, there is an incredible percentage of people in this country who might very well be on Medicaid who are not covered because of the varying eligibility rules, people who are being taken care of outside the system. We need a new set of numbers that accurately reflects the actual cost of medical care for these people.

What disturbs me is that we are now in the position of suddenly having the funds dry up. If we do not separate out all the nonmedical expenses in this system, we run a very real risk of destroying the system for the wrong reasons, and blaming the wrong people—with absolutely no replacement in sight. I think it is time to stop talking about this issue as though we really knew what Medicaid expenditures are, because I don't think we do.

Dr. Alan Nelson: One number that we have not been given, and I have never been able to get, is the amount spent administering Medicaid programs in comparison with the amount paid out in benefits. I have never heard anybody give a rational figure for that, although I once heard that in New York City the total expenditures to administer the program exceeded the number of dollars paid out in benefits. What is the administrative cost, as a percentage of the total expenditure?

Mr. Joseph A. Califano, Jr.: It is far less than 10 percent.

Professor Karen Davis: The administrative expense of Medicaid runs about 4 percent of benefits payments and that of Medicare is about 3 percent.

Dr. Nelson: The second point I want to make has to do with the extraordinary difficulty of determining eligibility. The Medicaid patient that I see is often not much different from his neighbor, except that the Medicaid patient has found out how to contact the social worker and get into the system and the neighbor not on Medicaid has found out how to get a job. Apart from that, there may not be a great deal of difference. Does anyone believe the federal government can conduct very difficult eligibility determinations more efficiently than the states?

The third point has to do with the fact that expenditures for Medicaid have been going up as the number of recipients has increased. Is that because there are more poor people, or is it because we have created a vast army of social workers whose jobs depend on identifying clients for the program?

Mr. Paul Rogers: The public is very much aware of many of these problems, and there are movements developing as a result of their concern. One alternative that may or may not turn out to be a solution to high costs is home health care. This is a new strategy that will have to be tested, but it may help to reduce the cost of caring for the elderly.

Support is also building among the public for changing the options about dying, for death with dignity; the hospice movement is one result. A lot of dying patients will still want expensive care, but this new idea is gaining strength to the point where reimbursement for terminal care in the hospice is possible.

These two alternatives are beginning to receive public support, and they may help to solve some of the problems of care for the aged.

Dr. E. Harvey Estes, Jr.: Most of the high costs associated with dying are incurred when older people no longer have control over their own decision making and others begin to make these decisions for them. As a result, some older people are now beginning to make these decisions ahead of time in the form of "living wills."

My second comment relates to the maintenance costs that Dr. Ginzberg mentioned, specifically nursing home expenditures. One of our Duke faculty members has done a lot of work with the rural elderly, and she finds that they have an almost universal aversion to institutionalization. The impetus for nursing home placement does not usually come from the older people; it comes from their families. The families are unwilling to assume the inconvenience and cost of their care. Maybe this can be changed by some administrative rule making. Another important point is that it is not in the best interest of elderly people to be institutionalized. Death is accelerated, not deterred, by institutionalization.

My third observation relates to total health care costs. An additional reason that we have seen so much attention paid to health care costs in the past five years is because health care must now compete more intensely with other systems for scarce dollars. The cost of every other service system (food, transportation, housing, etc.) has gone up too, largely because of higher energy costs. Everything costs more, and the competition grows more fierce.

Dr. Daniel C. Tosteson: The issue is not so much the extent to which we can reduce costs for the care of the elderly and the poor, but the extent to which we can contain the increase in expenditures that seem necessary. I appreciate the possibility that there is a lot of fat in the system, yet there seems to be a consensus that a lot of people are not now getting services they truly need. Somebody is going to have to pay for those services. Clearly, that means unit costs must be contained, which will require some kind of prospective budget in which contracts are made between providers and payers, both private and government sources. Doesn't this mean a return to a two-class—or more than one-class—system? Don't we need to be honest about the fact that this is going to happen and about its meaning? It is hard for me to believe that the unit costs for the care of the poor and the elderly can be kept the same as those for the rest of the population that can pay.

I wonder if Dr. Rogers would comment on the role of academic medical centers, teaching hospitals, and medical schools in all of this. Pre-Medicaid, there was a way of dealing with this issue, using the great municipal hospitals of this country. I am wondering whether some kind of cooperative approach between the academic medical centers, the private sector, and government could move us toward a new multi-class system that would be ethically tenable.

Dr. David Rogers: The innocence of the mid-sixties is gone. Unless we change our priorities I do not see how we can continue unfettered freedom-of-choice care for all of our citizens. It seems to me that we will inevitably retreat toward a two-class system. We have allowed the public part of our system to atrophy very badly, in part because of the way we have decided to finance health care. Major municipal hospitals are having a very difficult time. Mayors and governors would like to see them dry up and blow away. It will require quite a bit of retooling and rethinking to keep them solvent and functioning.

We must focus on the minority who continue to have a tough time getting medical care, not the majority. We will probably have to devise a system that takes care of those who are unable to take care of themselves.

Dr. Tosteson: It does not seem feasible to approach the problem exclusively or even primarily through the municipal hospitals. It has to be through the teaching hospitals and the private sector.

Dr. David Rogers: I agree.

Dr. C. Rollins Hanlon: I want to comment on a point raised by Dr. Ginzberg. He said, and I agree, that it is no secret that part of the high cost of dying comes from using patients, dying and recovering, as an educational testing ground for students, interns, and other house officers. This should not obscure the basic educational principle, which is that the best theoretical education is congruous with the most ethical and the most economical care of the patient.

Students and house officers should be told that it is wrong to do tests for their own sake or because this is the only chance they will get to do them before they get out in the world. That is bad education now, when costs are prodigious, and it is a bad principle.

Mr. Jack Shelton: My question, which involves the business community, has to do with the way we reimburse Medicaid and Medicare expenditures. The present reimbursement system entails a substantial cost shift, which may not be reflected in the numbers we see today. That is one of the reasons that the average cost for Medicaid eligibles is very close to the average cost for non-Medicaid eligibles. Because of the difficulty of adjusting eligibility requirements or changing the benefit structure, the easiest course for the government has always been to modify reimbursements—thus shifting to the private sector costs that are not reflected in total government expenditures for the programs. What troubles me is the negative reaction of the business community to increased costs of all kinds, including health care costs. In the auto industry, health costs are increasing at the same high rate as three or four years ago, and they are of great concern to management. Our costs in 1982, for example, are going to be almost $190 million higher than in 1979 despite our having 78,000 fewer active employees and 60,000 fewer insured.

Ms. Margaret Mahoney: One reason to discuss the elderly with the poor at this conference is because the number of elderly people who are poor is likely to grow substantially. This increase is of significant concern when one confronts the issues of designing programs and of determining how to pay for them. Dr. Ginzberg mentioned that 30 percent of Medicare expenditures are for patients in acute care facilities who are within twelve months of death. The anticipated increase in numbers of elderly people in the population means that the expenditures for hospital care during the last months of life will increase. So, looking for different and less expensive ways to take care of people at that stage of life becomes very important. Can we do some experiments to find ways of taking care of people in a different fashion at less expense? At the same time can we look at the consequences of moving dollars away from hospitals that depend on heavy use of their acute beds by the elderly.

Chairman William G. Anlyan: In the USSR they solved that by not admitting anybody over the age of eighty to an acute care hospital, but we can't do that here. In the United Kingdom they put you on a list, and you may die long before a hospital bed is available. This is a societal problem that we haven't found the right solution for in the United States.

Mr. Walter McNerney: Dr. Rogers made the point that as the government looked around for places to save money, two targets were Medicare and Medicaid. Of the two, Medicare seemed better protected. If Medicaid were run as well as Medicare, would the public feel the same skepticism about the program?

Dr. David Rogers: Not as much. Because of the politics of the situation, though, Medicaid would remain suspect in many ways, and it is a confusing program.

Mr. Califano: I think Medicaid is a far more complicated program to run. My empirical view is that everything we tried to do at HEW was geometrically harder when people thought we were doing it for black people, whether it was integrating a school, financing health care, or providing social services. If the beneficiaries were Hispanics or women we could move, but once people perceived that they were black it got harder. I think that fact hurt Medicaid far more than the perception that it is difficult to administer.

Dr. Richard Wilbur: One frequently expressed major concern is the increasing share of the Gross National Product devoted to health care. If living maintenance costs that are nonmedical were removed from this share, however, we would not have so serious a problem with the proportion of the Gross National Product devoted to health care. I state this as a serious proposition. We have been told that 75 percent of the 38 percent of Medicaid that is devoted to the elderly is spent for nursing home care. Very little of this is truly health care. If we were to substract maintenance costs, we would reduce the share of the Gross National Product devoted to health care. We would also highlight expenditures for nursing home care and ask why so many people have to be in nursing homes. Is there not something we can do in a social way, not only home health care, but home social care or home maintenance care, to reduce significantly this expenditure, which is increasing more and more rapidly? Then Medicaid expenses could be limited to expenditures for true health care.

I think that, when we compare the United States with other Western countries, we must make some allowance for the fact that a significant percentage of our population is from the Third World—from Mexico, from Haiti, from Vietnam and other parts of the world. These people do not have the same health and income statistics as those who have been here for more than a generation. I think that if we were able to examine the figures for the immigrant workers in Germany, or even in Sweden, we would find that their statistics are not as good as those of the native population either. Were we not still standing with open arms to the struggling, the poor, the masses, I think our health care statistics would be better. Whether we would be better people or not is another question. But we must allow for the fact that we are attempting to do something that other nations are not attempting to do.

Prof. David Mechanic: I think we have not even begun to see the tough problem, which is the balancing of developing technology on the one hand and demography on the other. When we talk about the problems of the last year of life, we are hearing the echoes of the values that the health professions have perpetuated. The professions have sold us on the "technological fix," and sold it so well that we insist on more and more technology. Indeed, despite all the increases in health care cost, most surveys show fantastic support among the general public for increased technology.

The problem is essentially a matter of social values, and the problem is going to get worse. How do we balance the competing interests? The major interests do not want to change. The hospitals want to go on as they have traditionally gone on; the physicians want to go on as they have gone on. We are at an impasse. Given the power of those two interests, we attack the weakest point: the poor and the elderly indigent, and the programs that serve them.

I am happy to see us attack the issue of maintenance costs, but it is very important when we talk about care for old people that we talk about the trade-offs between medical care and social medical care. One has to keep in mind the need to provide good social medical care and the need to feed all those physicians coming down the pipeline, who were trained to pursue technology during a time of constrained resources. I think that is the challenge and the problem.

Mr. Califano: We should not forget that the rising costs of the public programs are increasingly a measure of the interest groups getting money from those programs. For example, most of the processing of Medicare and Medicaid claims is done by insurance companies and intermediaries. When Medicare and Medicaid were passed, they and the hospitals fought hard for and got a provision which said that the government could not bid competitively, but that it had to take the provider the hospital wanted. When I became secretary, and that was brought to my attention by a businessman who wanted to bid, I found that competitive bidding would cause the American Hospital Association and the Blues to sue. It is not government regulation that has turned the reimbursement situation into a tax code; it is the people who are on the receiving end.

I currently sit on the Chrysler board, chairing a health care committee for the directors. Our committee went out to find which medical procedure our insurance carriers were paying the most for, and we found that medical procedure to be the bedside visit after the patient is operated on by the doctor. That is the single largest amount of money the Chrysler Corporation's insurance company is paying for physician services for its employees. We all know the reality of that situation, and we have to deal with that side of the table as well as the government side of the table.

Mr. Joseph N. Onek: I sympathize with Dr. Rogers' concern for physicians who do not want to play God. Their training does not really equip them to decide whether to spend $10,000 for a 1 percent chance of improving or increasing life expectancy. Nor can you put the burden on the patient, who in many cases is too far gone to make that decision. And, increasingly in our atomistic society, the family either does not exist or is not available.

We should probably be thinking about whether there are not some other kinds of institutions, informal ones, perhaps voluntary peer review, that can take the burden off individual physicians. In some cases it would take the burden off family members also, because it is very difficult to decide whether continued high intensity treatment in the hospital is necessary or whether a hospice or other alternative would be better. I do not think we can put the entire burden on the physicians, and I doubt very much that we can place it all on the patients or their families.

With respect to the Medicaid program, we have to recognize that there are going to be changes and that we are going to move toward a two-tier system. One matter that I hope we might address is the question of reneging from the freedom-of-choice ideals of the Medicaid program. Could we insist that only certain institutions be used by Medicaid patients, whether municipal hospitals or academic health centers in urban areas? What would be the sacrifices and what might be the potential gains? Can we sacrifice the principle of freedom of choice without sacrificing health care quality?

Dr. John A. D. Cooper: I want to make two comments. One is that we do not know the total cost of the care of the poor or the aged. The Council of Teaching Hospitals of the AAMC, whose members make up about 5 percent of the hospitals in the country, provide about 25 to 30 percent of charity care and 25 to 30 percent of bad debt care. By shifting the costs of that care to private payers, they have relieved the pressure on governments at every level to increase expenditures for the care of the poor and the aged.

The second point I would like to make is that when you refer to the question of the percentage of the GNP that is expended for health care, you have a numerator and a denominator. We always talk about the numerator: how much are we spending for health care? We don't talk about the denominator, the GNP, which has increased very slowly lately. One reason the ratio of health care expenses to GNP increases is the fact that the denominator has not increased at the traditional rate in this country.

Dr. John E. Affeldt: Dr. Anlyan made reference to the utilization controls employed in Russia and England. I am reminded of the time when the English would not build hospitals because that would mean beds were not available. That was another form of controlling utilization.

Before Medicaid we had a public system in municipal and county hospitals, with a built-in utilization control at the admitting point. Physicians had to choose the patients they would admit because there was room only for the critically ill. That, too, was a form of utilization control. There has been no utilization control under Medicaid, except by PSRO, and that was not very effective.

Dr. Tom E. Nesbitt: When Medicaid came into existence, a number of us at this conference served on our various state Medicaid advisory committees, struggling with limited resources to define benefit packages and to channel those resources in ways that would meet the medical care needs of the poor. Despite our conscientious efforts, we have seen those benefit packages altered, with the result that half the dollars are now channeled into long-term care, which we did not perceive to be the real aim of the Medicaid program.

A conference that is convened to talk about the care of the elderly and the poor is really talking about three separate elements: (1) medical care for the poor, (2) medical care for the elderly, and (3) long-term care for the elderly. Fifty years from now there will be 50 million Americans over the age of sixty-five. That is why it is imperative that we separate the need for *long-term* care of the elderly from the *medical* care needs of the elderly and from the medical care needs of the poor. We could begin by defining the elderly. Is it those who are not employed, or those who have had a certain birthday, or those who are disabled?

A comment about the cost of medical care: I have long been concerned that the physician population gets the credit for making the decisions that result in the expenditure of about 70 to 72 percent of the $247 billion spent on medical care in 1981. If the physicians in this country have that great an impact on the system, what can we, as concerned professionals and business people and economists, do to modify their behavior pattern? Where do we begin to create an understanding of the need to modify their behavior pattern? Do we begin at medical school? Do we begin at the hospital staff level? Do we begin with trade associations? Or do we have to wait until a regulatory arm of government imposes that type of decision-making process? Recognizing that the behavior pattern of physicians is a major problem to be addressed, what do we do with the coming expansion in the supply of physicians?

Mr. John W. Colloton: There have been suggestions that we use less expensive types of personnel, restrain the use of high-cost technology, further constrain care to the terminally ill, and even return to the two-class system. My question is: how do we do all this within present legal and regulatory boundaries? Our legal system is constantly pushing for higher standards of practice, while licensing laws and regulations for hospitals are becoming ever more pervasive. Current funding reductions have not been accompanied by exemptions from these pressures. They seem instead to give providers three options: first, to refuse to provide care; second, to continue rendering it at a substantial and growing loss; third, to render it under a two-class system at our own risk. If academic medical centers are to structure a discrete system for care of the elderly and the poor and survive financially, we need some relief in the area of legal and regulatory constraints.

Dr. Sammons: Two words have been noticeably absent from our dialogue thus far: want and demand. Regardless of our individual perspectives, we must take into account patient wants, patient demands, and societal demands. One of the most frightening numbers that I have run across in a long time is that half of all of the people who have lived to reach the age of sixty-five since the beginning of recorded history are living today! If we do not take into account what those people expect for themselves, especially as they become a progressively larger segment of our society, we are not going to solve the problem.

There seems to be a popular conception that medicine is not changing and doctors are not changing. Nothing could be further from the truth! Our studies show change at work in medicine. There are 156,000 doctors in this country today who have some kind of financial relationship with a hospital, many more than ever before. There are 90,000 physicians practicing in medical groups in this country, and that number is increasing rapidly. We are beginning to see a redistribution of physicians, partly because of the economic downturn in the cities and the highly competitive nature of a city practice. We are beginning to see reductions in the sizes of the classes in medical schools. We are seeing some very early signs of marked change. Until we start putting into this dialogue the terms "want" and "demand," however, we are not going to solve the problems. The public will solve this problem in its own good time. We are either going to have to help them decide how to solve it, or they will do it without us. We will either have to do it as a profession or abdicate it to government.

Dr. Roscoe R. Robinson: There are some things forcing a solution that are a consequence of recognizable market forces and the impact of reimbursement regulations. Among the solutions presently being forced upon us are a return to the two-tier system, denial of care, and rationing of care. I represent an academic health center that has taken pride in the fact that, in its entire history, it has not denied care to any of those who have come to its doors. Recent cost shifting has become so great, though, that for the first time the institution has been obliged to deny or limit care to the poor. I suspect that we are also sitting in another institution that may be examining the same kinds of considerations. This constraint on services to the poor is an interesting consequence of two things: the impact of federal reimbursement regulations, and the impact of market forces on those who can afford to pay. The latter are saying that there has been more than enough cost shifting. There can be no more—and the consequence is a denial of care to those very people whom the initial legislation was intended to serve.

Dr. David Rogers: I would like to respond to Dr. Nesbitt. He asked whether it is time for the provider group, primarily physicians, who are the major generators of costs, to come together to responsibly downsize the system. My response is that I am very encouraged that it is indeed time.

There is no reason why physicians cannot put together a tribal council that the profession would recognize and respect to see what can be done. One thing that encourages me is that now there seem to be some ways of putting guidelines in place for physicians. I did not think that was possible before.

I have recently looked with some care at the ways NIH has used their consensus panels. I also talked with Dr. Donald Fredrickson during his tenure as Director of the NIH. I am beginning to see where a thoughtful group of professionals could indeed say: "These are some reasonable guidelines to make more discriminating and more restrained use of the dollars in the system which can protect fellow physicians who feel exposed and alone because there are no professionally developed guidelines." It seems that a great deal could be done in that area, and I sense a willingness on the part of the medical profession to try and do it.

Dr. Ginzberg: I would agree with Dr. Sammons that the system is changing rapidly. It will change much more rapidly because of its uncontrollable parts. So far we have identified only two of those parts: a large increase in the number of physicians and a reduction in the number of easy dollars.

I would forecast a major competitive struggle between physicians and hospitals in the years immediately ahead. The only way that physicians can decelerate the rate at which their incomes will go down is to shift money from institutions to themselves. Having said that, I expect to see a major reduction in the size, scale, and level of operations of hospitals, reversing the trend of the 1960s and 1970s. During the last twenty years, physicians and hospitals have worked together because it was a mutually satisfactory arrangement. I expect to see just the opposite now. The chief surgeon of a major teaching hospital in New York says he can do 30 percent of his surgery outside the hospital. Now for the first time, there are going to be strong incentives for him to do it.

I always thought we had two levels of health care during the years we had Medicaid. I believe we will have more of that.

I also think Dr. Robinson is right. We will begin to see rationing and denial of care and admissions. A journalist from Montreal told me recently that the Canadian system is so paralyzed that in Montreal they cannot operate the emergency room anymore because the hospitals are so full. They cannot simply discharge their long-term patients, and so they are unable to admit anyone into the emergency room.

With respect to the aged, one of our problems is that we do not know how to distinguish between maintenance care, health care, institutional care, and community care. The critical issue is whether any of the new alternatives, such as home care, are going to be supplemental or substitutive. Are they substitutive? We do not know yet. On the basis of my study for Blue Cross in New York, I am afraid they will add to cost, not reduce it. It will take very tight management to make them substitutive.

I would end by saying that I think we have not defined as sharply as we should the things that we wish to make clear to people in Washington and in the state capitals. We need to decide which few issues are so important that they should be carefully researched. How much do we understand the changing market out there? The consumer? The forces operating powerfully beneath the surface?

Session II

5. The Challenge to the Health Care System: Can the Third Biggest Business Take Care of the Medically Indigent? A Personal Perspective

Joseph A. Califano, Jr.

Health is our second largest employer (behind education) and our third largest industry in consumer spending (after food and housing), and it is growing faster than any other. Federal, state, and local governments are by far the largest purchasers of health care. Unchecked, the health industry is more likely to consume Americans' private and public dollars than the oil sheiks. In 1980, Americans spent two dollars on health care for each dollar they spent on oil.

In 1965 Americans spent $39 billion, 5.9 percent of their Gross National Product, on health care. By 1980, Americans were spending about $230 billion, more than 9 percent. That amounts to a levy of $1,000 on each man, woman, and child in America, and the average employed American worked more than a month in 1980 to pay it. The average family spends more than 12 percent of its income for health care. Private health insurance premiums have been rising at about 18 percent a year during the past several years. Hospital charges—the fastest rising costs in the health industry—have climbed more rapidly than the consumer price index, from 1975 to 1978 rising at more than twice the general rate of inflation, pausing briefly under the threat of federal cost-containment legislation, and promptly resuming their steep annual hikes as soon as that threat receded. By the year 2000, under the present system, Americans will turn over at least $1 trillion—12 percent of the Gross National Product—to the health care industry.

Almost seven million people are employed in the health industry, about 7 percent of the national work force, one American worker out of every fourteen. And the trend is up: from 1970 to 1978, employment in the industry increased by 60 percent, accounting for one out of every seven new jobs created. Almost 450,000 physicians practice, and about 1.5 million nurses assist them. There are more than 7,000 hospitals, with a capacity of 1.4 million beds, and more than 18,000 skilled nursing homes with another 1.4 million beds. Thousands of laboratories, hundreds of suppliers of drugs, expensive medical equipment, and all sorts of medical products and devices, and a growing army of insurance salesmen, claims processors, home health aides, and nonprofessionals in hospitals and nursing homes make their living in the health care industry.

In 1965 HEW's health budget was $1.9 billion. Fifteen years later, with Medicare and Medicaid, it was $55 billion. Payments under Medicare have risen geometrically to fund increasingly expensive equipment and procedures and the health problems that accompany the aging of America's population. In 1980, about fifteen cents of every tax dollar spent was paid to the health industry.

The investment of tax dollars has brought significant advances in access to quality health care. In 1980, Medicare paid $34 billion in health care bills for 28 million elderly and disabled Americans. Since Medicare began, life expectancy for the elderly has increased by almost two years; days lost from work by the elderly have decreased by 50 percent. Millions of senior citizens have access to health care only because of the program. In 1980, Medicaid paid $24.5 billion ($14.2 billion, federal; $10.3 billion, state) for the health care of 23 million poor people. During the first ten years of Medicaid, death rates from diseases that are historically prevalent among the poor declined sharply: infant mortality rates were down by 33 percent and maternal mortality rates by 66 percent; death rates from influenza and pneumonia dropped by 28 percent and from strokes by 30 percent. The use of preventive services by the poor has increased since Medicaid: the proportion of poor women who receive early pregnancy care from a physician rose from 17 percent in 1963 to 65 percent in 1976; the number of physician visits per year by poor children climbed by 26 percent from 1964 to 1979.

While Medicare and Medicaid have helped improve access and the health status of millions of elderly and poor Americans, they have also contributed to the inflation, inefficiency, and waste that have persistently characterized the health care industry. Despite the explosion of the health care industry over the 1970s, 50 million people live in areas with severe shortages of health personnel services. However unlikely any sort of national health plan may be, it is imperative to provide health care to the 20 million poor Americans presently not covered by Medicaid and to close gaps in coverage for the elderly, disabled, and poor already receiving benefits.

Inflation, Inefficiency, and Waste

The health business is not inflationary, inefficient, and wasteful because doctors and hospital administrators wear black hats while patients wear white ones. By and large, doctors and hospital administrators respond to the economic incentives and penalties they face just as most people in the business world do. Most patients do not give sufficient attention to their hospital and doctor bills because they're not paying them directly. Under the third-party reimbursement system, more than 90 percent of all hospital bills and 66 percent of doctor bills are paid by Medicare, Medicaid, other government programs, or insurance companies. By contrast, fifty years ago 90 percent of all health care bills were paid by individuals. Not paying the bill directly, few patients relate it to their health insurance premiums or taxes. Those who do conclude that asking doctors about costs and bills or questioning the need for particular services will have no impact on their own insurance premiums or tax payments. And millions of

Americans do not pay anything for health insurance—employers or the government picks up the bill.

In business transactions there is normally a direct relationship between buyers and sellers and competition. When an American buys a television set or a car, he chooses the dealer and pays for his purchase directly. He discusses the price with the salesman, picks the model he wants, and selects the optional features he wants.

But there is no such direct relationship between buyer and seller, and virtually no competition among sellers, in the health care industry. The patient may select a family doctor, but rarely the specialist, the hospital, the surgery, the often expensive medical tests. Nobody walks into a hospital and asks for an appendectomy, hysterectomy, or coronary bypass. The doctor determines which medical procedures are required, and he doesn't pay the bill.

The third-party reimbursement system and the lack of competition have helped to perpetuate expensive methods of charging for health care. Almost all health care bills are paid on a fee-for-service or cost-plus basis. The more services that are rendered, the more fees we pay. When an American goes to a doctor or hospital, the financial incentive is for the provider to supply the services. The fee-for-service system offers little financial incentive for health promotion and disease prevention or for curing a sick patient at the lowest cost with the fewest services.

Moreover, the incentives and penalties encourage providing the most expensive services. Insurance covers hospital and acute care far more extensively than preventive care, such as periodical physical exams or immunizations. The possibility of malpractice litigation prompts physicians to perform unnecessary tests to protect themselves against accusations of negligence.

The absence of competition, the lack of buyer-seller tension, and the third-party and fee-for-service reimbursement systems turn the traditional concept of free enterprise on its head. The more doctors, nursing homes, and hospitals we have, the more expensive the system gets. The more specialists there are, the more referrals to specialists there are; the more equipment a hospital has, the more tests it runs on its patients. These greater expenses turn into higher health insurance premiums, higher bills from doctors, hospitals, and laboratories, and higher prices of products to recoup the more expensive employee health benefits. These higher costs in turn require higher taxes to support the biggest buyer of goods and services from America's health care colossus—the federal, state, and local governments that pay 54 percent of all hospital bills.

State and municipal health departments have traditionally committed significant resources to health care, including the operation of hospitals and public health services. Since World War II, substantial federal money has been directed to the health care system through the Veterans Administration (particularly in recent years, with the aging of World War II veterans), the Defense Department, and the federal employee health plans. But the greatest single infusion of federal funds came during the Great Society years of the mid-1960s when, at the insistent urging of President Lyndon Johnson, Congress passed forty health bills. There was a need to increase the access of our people to health care. We responded with funds to pay the bills where need was most severe. To increase our ability to provide such care, we provided resources to expand enrollments in medical and nursing schools, and to build more hospitals. We had hoped that a more plentiful supply of doctors, nurses, and hospitals would curtail sharp cost increases due to the demand our programs would create.

For senior citizens over age sixty-five and for the disabled, the Great Society put together Medicare, a completely federal program financed largely out of Social Security payroll taxes. For the poor—"the medically needy" as the federal regulations call them—we established Medicaid, a program funded jointly by the federal government and the states, with the wide flexibility for each state to define "medically needy" and to determine what health care services it would fund, in what proportion, and at what rate.

President Johnson was keenly aware of the potential of the Medicaid program to help poor people. There was no focus on it in Congress, no testimony, and no hearings for one simple reason: the President was convinced that it would be perceived, as it has been, as a program for black people and that it would never get through Congress. The political arrangement was to keep Medicaid out of the Social Security system so that senior citizen groups would support it.

In the often bitter struggles to get Medicare and Medicaid enacted, the focus was almost entirely on access, rarely on cost. Sitting in Johnson's small green hideaway adjoining the Oval Office one day, White House congressional lobbyists Larry O'Brien and Wilbur Cohen (later to become HEW Secretary) responded to Johnson's demand that they move the Medicare bill out of committee. "It'll cost a half-billion dollars to make the changes in reimbursement standards to get the bill out of the Senate Finance Committee," Cohen said.

"Five hundred million. Is that all?" Johnson exclaimed with a wave of his big hand. "Do it. Move that damn bill out now, before we lose it."

The opposition to Medicare by the health industry—insurance companies, hospitals, and particularly doctors—was so unyielding that in 1965 we were concerned whether sufficient numbers of doctors would participate. By the time I became HEW Secretary in 1977, the doctors' reluctance, like that of other providers, had given way to their heavy involvement, with complaints only about filling out forms and publishing the fees participating physicians received from Medicare and Medicaid. Doctors and others were being paid billions of dollars by the two programs for whatever procedures doctors considered "medically necessary" in Medicare on the basis of their "reasonable cost and customary charges." Health insurance agencies and computer companies processed millions of claims each month for federal and state governments. The sapling nursing home business of the early 1960s had grown to a $22 billion forest, as forty cents of each Medicaid dollar went into its coffers. (Today in most states the number has risen to fifty cents.) Medicare guaranteed income to hospitals and profits to the high-technology medical equipment industry, often funding exotic and expensive means to extend life under extraordinary circumstances. Twenty-five percent of Medicare's $34 billion budget in 1980 was spent on care rendered during the last year of life. With too few exceptions, Medicare reimbursed hospitals for whatever costs they incurred, and whatever expensive equipment they purchased, no matter how infrequently it was used.

By 1977 the once diehard opponents of Medicare and Medicaid—the health insurers, hospital administrators, and doctors—were enjoying supping at the public table. In its rush to provide access, the Great Society had let the health industry set the prices and had acquiesced in its reimbursement systems. Over the intervening decade, the industry had used America's quest for broad access to quality health care to protect and enhance its financial interest and to solidify its legislative and regulatory position. The health industry was seated comfortably at a groaning table set by the taxpayers.

Administrative Difficulties of Medicare and Medicaid

A key to persuading Congress to provide additional health care benefits to the poor, particularly children and the elderly, was to demonstrate that the existing Medicare and Medicaid programs could be operated efficiently. Our reorganization of Medicare and Medicaid into a single Health Care Financing agency and the creation of the new Inspector General Office gave us an opportunity to mount major efforts to eliminate fraud, abuse, and waste in the government health programs. The effort was critical for an administration that was asking for a major expansion of Medicaid to cover child health and prenatal care, and for a national health plan. Since Medicare and Medicaid involved millions of transactions each month, we used computers as policemen. We followed up with selective criminal prosecutions in each state so that the publicity would help deter future offenders.

Medicare is a single program, operated by the federal government through insurance and computer companies that process claims for payment. Individual eligibility is easy to determine: all those over sixty-five years of age and all receiving Social Security disability payments. The kinds of treatment covered are uniform nationally. Less than 1 percent of Medicare funds for the elderly are erroneously spent for ineligible individuals or to pay for health care services not covered by the program.

By contrast, in 1980 Medicaid was fifty-three different health plans—one for each state (except Arizona, which had not adopted it), the District of Columbia, and the territories. Each jurisdiction set its own income level for determining eligible individuals or families. Each has wide discretion to establish the health care services that will be covered and the portion of the charge that will be reimbursed. The millions of Medicaid transactions that occur in this complex administrative environment are prone to error and abuse. Much of the waste in Medicaid is a result of its inherent complexity. Determinations of eligibility turn on such fine points that it is not possible to train thousands of individuals to administer the program with accuracy. But the potential of computers to improve payment efficiency and accuracy was enormous, and we pressed states and cities to establish sophisticated computer systems.

In 1976 and 1977 the proportion of funds paid for individuals or medical procedures not entitled to reimbursement ranged as high as 49 percent in the District of Columbia, with several states hovering around 25 percent. With the use of computers and other quality control techniques, by 1979 we were able to cut the District of Columbia's error rate to 24 percent and to reduce the states' error rates to an average just below 10 percent—significant improvements, but still unacceptably high.

When a sophisticated computer system was installed in New York City in 1978, we immediately began saving millions of dollars each month, largely by eliminating duplicate payments. Some duplicate bills were fraudulent, but most were customary thirty- or sixty-day notices for unpaid bills that older billing systems had never rejected after the original bill was paid. By paying most bills within two weeks, these computer systems provided another benefit: they encouraged doctors to accept Medicaid patients. Because payments for services for Medicaid patients are lower than for other patients and because of the increased paperwork required to recoup late payments, it had become increasingly difficult to enlist doctors to serve Medicaid patients. In New York City when we introduced the computer system with its prompt payments we doubled in a year the number of physicians willing to take Medicaid patients.

Our problems with Medicaid fraud were serious and led to the development in April 1977 of one of our most ingenious computer detective systems, Project Integrity. Initially we deployed Project Integrity against Medicaid doctors and pharmacists. For physicians, we identified twenty-two common medical procedures, from office visits to hysterectomies, and established an outside number of times each procedure might be performed on an individual in a year. For example, we set four visits for a patient to a doctor's office as the outside limit. Obviously, more than one appendectomy on an individual patient was impossible. For pharmacists, we established outside limits for twenty-six commonly prescribed drugs. More than twenty-five prescriptions for Valium in a single year for one patient was deemed unreasonable.

We then ran computer tapes of the Medicaid procedures for each doctor and patient and the Medicaid prescriptions for each pharmacist and customer against our outside limits. For 1976—the first year against which we deployed these computer screens—we identified more than 47,000 physicians and pharmacists who had exceeded the outside limits.

Stunned by their number, we narrowed the list down to about five hundred cases in each state. With the state usually taking the lead, we conducted an investigation to determine the circumstances surrounding the raw computer hit, and then selected the most serious case involving twenty-five physicians and twenty-five druggists in each jurisdiction. At first it was difficult to interest U.S.

attorneys and state prosecuters in pursuing doctors and pharmacists for what they regarded as very small crimes.

Federalizing Medicaid

With effective computer policing and management, the Medicare program can be run at a high level of efficiency; Medicaid, however, is more complicated. The most sophisticated electronic and management techniques will significantly reduce the payments for ineligible patients or ineligible procedures, but they are not likely to achieve a program with error rates as low as Medicare. Only with major legislative surgery, such as federalization or at least uniform eligibility standards for individuals and medical procedures, will Medicaid operate efficiently. A federal takeover of the financing and operation of Medicaid may find increasing political support, as in more and more states it consumes a larger share of tax dollars than welfare.

What the Reagan administration appears to be proposing as part of its "New Federalism" program in the fiscal 1983 budget seems less a true federal assumption of Medicaid than the wolf of budget cutting in the sheep's clothing of federalization.

First, the principal keys to the door to Medicaid benefits are eligibility for Aid to Families with Dependent Children (about 8 million mothers, 3 million children and perhaps 500,000 fathers) and Supplemental Security Income (the poor, aged, disabled, and blind). The gaps in coverage of poor people are significant; for example, AFDC does not cover pregnant women who are not already mothers. Several million poor people who are not eligible for these welfare programs should be covered as part of any serious federalization of Medicaid. The poor, and particularly minorities, pay a frightful price for lack of access to health care, as well as for poverty. The life expectancy of a black man in the United States is only age sixty-four, below the Social Security retirement age and eight years below life expectancy for a white man, and a black woman is two times more likely than a white woman to lose her infant or her own life in childbirth.

Second, benefits covered by states vary enormously. Serious federalization should bring all benefits closer to the comprehensive coverage of states like California and New York, rather than low-benefit states like Mississippi and Tennessee. Medicaid is particularly tilted toward acute care rather than health promotion and disease prevention. Federalization should encourage health promotion and disease prevention.

Third, and in many ways most important, federalization of Medicaid should encourage major system reforms in reimbursement and delivery of health care. In the interest of simplified administration, federalization should have the ultimate objective of making Medicare and Medicaid a single program. This relates not only to forms and other administrative paraphernalia, but also to the level of payment and the procedures covered.

Fourth, one of the principles should be copayment by those who can afford it. Recent Rand studies indicate that copayments are indeed important. Those who can afford to pay part of their health care costs should be required to do so.

The Reagan plan seems unlikely to correct any of these deficiencies. As projected in its budget, Medicaid benefits would be cut by $2 billion (from $19 to $17 billion) in 1983, and more in later years. That doesn't take inflation into account; health care programs can easily go up at twice the rate of the consumer price index. So Reagan's 1983 federalization proposal may in reality represent a $4 billion cut for Medicaid. Other programs that assist poor people are also being cut—most notably childhood immunization, community health, and a host of grants, particularly in areas like alcoholism, drug abuse, and maternal and child health care. Many categories of grants can be consolidated, but cutting their funding is shortsighted. In the long run, cuts in Medicaid and other health programs for the poor guarantee a far more costly health care bill, in addition to the human suffering such cuts visit on the poor.

In the short run, reducing federal funds available to provide health care for the poor will increase the burden on public hospitals and private health insurers. Public hospitals are already overburdened, in some cases to the point of near-bankruptcy. Their emergency rooms in large urban areas receive more than twice the visits of large university hospitals and four times those of large urban private hospitals. In our large cities, public hospitals represent only 1.6 percent of the hospital beds, but they provide one-fourth of outpatient clinic services. Grady Memorial in Atlanta, for example, accounts for 53 percent of all clinic visits and 12.5 percent of all emergency room visits in the entire state of Georgia. These public hospitals have fifty fewer full-time equivalent staff per 100 patient days than other hospitals of comparable size, and thirty fewer than the average private hospitals.

To the extent public hospitals cannot pick up the added patient load, private hospitals will have to increase the share of indigent patients they care for. The reluctance of these hospitals to do so (with the notable exception of many university facilities) is notorious. But to the extent they do so now, those paying insurance premiums will have to ante up more money to cover the cost. In this sense the Reagan Administration proposal is less a thoughtful health plan than a transfer of the tax burden to states, cities, and insured patients.

Professional Resources and the Needs of the Indigent

If we are to truly care for the indigent among us, we need more primary care physicians than we are now producing. In September 1980 the Graduate Medical Education National Advisory Committee (GMENAC), headed by Dr. Alvin R. Tarlov of the University of Chicago's School of Medicine, concluded that, unchecked, the supply of active physicians will increase to 536,000 by 1990, providing 200 doctors for each 100,000 people in this country. The result will be a substantial oversupply of physicians: an excess of 70,000. The expected entry into practice over the next ten years of 40,000 to 50,000 graduates of foreign medical schools accounts for much of the surplus. By the year 2000, there will be an estimated 630,000 physicians, 130,000 more than we will need to serve our population.

The potential oversupply of doctors does not add to our ability to care for poor people because of two other characteristics: lopsided geographical distribution and overspecialization.

More money is not likely to lure more physicians to rural areas or inner cities. England, Germany, Italy, Israel, Canada, and Poland have the same problem, and none of those countries has been able to attract doctors to rural areas, even with bonuses, extra vacations, and special housing privileges. Only some kind of conscription has worked. In the United States, only the National Health Service Corps—a program that pays medical school tuition in return for a service commitment—has gotten doctors to rural areas.

To ease the geographic maldistribution problem, we almost tripled the size of the National Health Service Corps, from 725 in 1977 to 2,100 in 1980, and the number of HEW-funded community health centers, from 302 to 876. Through Medicaid demonstrations and Public Health Service programs, we worked with states and local communities to construct clinics in rural areas and to mount special efforts in inner cities, such as Harlem in New York. The cuts effected and proposed in the National Health Service Corps and these other programs will aggravate the maldistribution of physicians.

The other aspect of maldistribution is the concentration of physicians in expensive, lucrative specialties. As the specialties and subspecialties have proliferated, there has been a decline in the number of primary-care physicians who practice in pediatrics and internal and family medicine. These doctors should be the first point of contact between the patient and the health care system. They should provide as much of the health care as they can, referring the patient to more expensive specialists only when necessary.

In 1931 some 94 percent of American physicians were involved in primary care. By 1975 that figure had plummeted to 38 percent, compared with 72 percent in West Germany and 60 percent in Canada—and compared with the 50 percent minimum set by the American Association of Medical Colleges. If we continue as we have, only 35 to 40 percent of new physicians will enter the primary-care fields, and the already severe distortions in our physician profile will be exacerbated. There are some indications that the trend may be turning, but not yet sufficiently to fill our needs for primary-care physicians. And these are the ones poor people need most.

Health Promotion and Disease Prevention

From my earliest analysis of the HEW health budget, I understood what Hubert Humphrey meant when he said, "We have a system of sick care in this country, not health care." Of the almost $50 billion the federal government was spending on health care in 1977, almost 96 percent was aimed at treatment rather than programs to prevent disease or promote health.

The future of decent health care for all needy people rests more with health promotion and disease protection than with acute care. Our nation's first public health revolution was the struggle against infectious diseases from the late nineteenth to the mid-twentieth century. We won that battle not with cures, but with sanitation programs, pasteurization of milk, a safer food supply, the development of vaccines, and mass immunization. As a result, today only 1 percent of deaths before age seventy-five are from infectious diseases. In 1900, those diseases—influenza, pneumonia, diphtheria, tuberculosis, dysentery, and the like—were the leading cause of death.

Today heart disease, stroke, and cancer account for 70 percent of all deaths, and accidents exact a fearsome toll of disability as well as death from young Americans. Victory in the struggle against these killers lies more securely in prevention than in cure. That is also the less costly way to mount a second revolution in public health. Our scientists and physicians are developing the knowledge to win. But this battle is fraught with sharp controversy and demands a commitment of political and individual will we have yet to demonstrate.

Any major effort to promote health involves scientific and economic ingredients, financial incentives, and individual self-discipline. A cleaner environment, better drinking water, safe and nutritious food, elimination of carcinogens in food additives, and occupational health and safety standards (20 percent of cancer incidence is associated with chemicals in the workplace), for example, are all worthy objectives; but achievement of each in concrete situations is likely to provoke scientific disputes and to enhance or endanger specific economic interests. Changing financial incentives—such as convincing insurance companies and passing federal legislation to cover periodic physical exams, expanding reimbursement under government programs for physical rehabilitation, and paying doctors on other than a fee-for-service basis—is no task for the timid. There is a role for schools, yet introducing antismoking and sex-education programs in local school systems can often not be done without sharp conflict. But nowhere does controversy reach more intense levels, and nowhere is action more important, than in the area that is the key to health and the centerpiece of any health promotion and disease prevention program—personal life-style. Americans can do more for their own health than any doctors, any machine or hospital, by adopting healthy life-styles, but doing so relates to a host of personal habits, such as smoking, alcohol consumption, diet, exercise, sleep, and stress reduction. In a free society the role of government in this area is largely limited to informing and persuading people.

Morever, even informing and persuading can become controversial when you run up against powerful financial interests, and few are more powerful than the cigarette lobby. The cigarette industry sells a product that has killed more Americans more painfully—through heart disease, lung cancer, and choking to death from emphysema—than have all our wars and all our traffic accidents combined. The industry has often successfully blocked government attempts to educate our people to the life-threatening aspect of smoking. And a disproportionate number of the victims are the economically disadvantaged.

A General, Personal Reflection

As I reflect on my own experience with the nation's health care system, I am convinced that as a matter of intellect and management we can devise a national health care plan that the government can administer, particularly if we take advantage of the employer-employee relationship, direct the reimbursement system to reward health promotion and disease prevention, and mount massive health education efforts. Such a plan would carry the additional cost of providing proper health care to millions of Americans who do not presently have access to that care. But I believe that a well-crafted plan with the right mix of reforms in health care delivery, reimbursement incentives, and controls would cost less for each dollar of health care delivered than the present system with its rampant waste and social injustices.

Two other nagging considerations, however, have tempered my ardor and led me to hope the private sector can do more in health care and containing costs. So long as the congressional system is as vulnerable to special-interest groups as it now is, I doubt that we have the political independence and integrity in the Congress to enact a sound national health plan. The doctors, specialists, hospitals, nurses, unions, medical equipment suppliers, pharmaceutical industry, insurance and computer companies, medical schools, and others will all demand and get significant concessions as part of any national health program. By the time they do, the resulting legislation is likely to carve in the marble of the U.S. statutes many of the least effective and most costly and wasteful elements of the present system. Without substantial changes in the structure and process of the Congress, I believe that we are incapable of enacting a health plan that will serve the national interest.

The other concern that leads me to hope the private sector can do more is the ethical aspect of any national health plan. If our experience as a nation with federal funding of abortion provides any lessons, one surely is that federal funding of medical procedures instantly politicizes them and throws them into litigation. Ethical issues are arising in a host of other areas: psychosurgery, sterilization, the deployment of billions of taxpayer dollars for extraordinary life-extending equipment and services, the rights of terminally ill patients to try any cure—or to choose none. If the federal government funds—or mandates the funding of—most health services, it becomes the political battleground for all the ethical issues related to them. We need more experience and wisdom than we have yet displayed to learn how to cope fairly with these ethical issues in our national government. At this stage, I believe both freedom and morality are better served by leaving these decisions to a variety of individuals, doctors, hospitals, and communities than by asking the Secretary of Health and Human Services to play Solomon.

These two considerations—the ability of the special interests to manipulate the legislative process to consolidate existing economic advantages and achieve new ones, and the difficulty of dealing with the ethical issues in the political arena or in the courtroom—lead me to believe that we should move cautiously on any national health plan. This seems especially persuasive if we can find a way to increase pressure on the private sector to control health care costs.

We must, as a matter of social justice, provide health care to the millions of poor and unprotected Americans, particularly children and minorities. There are significant improvements to be made by federalizing Medicaid into a single program, opening up Medicare and Medicaid to more competition, putting a lid on hospital costs, encouraging more efficient delivery of health care services through health maintenance organizations and nurse practitioners, and moving the focus of our system from acute care to health promotion and disease prevention.

A few ideas:

First, the fundamental problem in our society is the economy. If we could get the economy working, an enormous number of our people and a large number of our problems would be taken care of.

Second, the role of the private sector in health promotion and disease prevention has not even been scratched. Employers are notorious for not taking care of their employees in a paternalistic way. Less than 12 percent of the employees in the United States work for employers who have anything resembling an employee assistance program directed at alcoholism, and alcoholism is now one of the top four diseases in the United States of America. Everybody here knows that the private sector, indeed the private nonmedical sector, can probably do more about that than anybody is going to do in the acute care system.

Third, business and labor can do a lot more to press insurance companies to hold premiums down and, in turn, to press hospitals and doctors to be more prudent about length of stay in the hospital and the ordering of tests.

Fourth, I don't think it is realistic in 1982 to have a retirement age of sixty-five. Clearly, the retirement age should be moved up to seventy. It is politics which makes that so difficult. I would make major changes in the way the elderly are cared for. I think, increasingly, they must be cared for in the home. It is worth looking at tax credits for children to take care of their parents.

Home health care is another important avenue. But, in addition to all the other problems that Dr. Ginzberg has mentioned with respect to home health care, it is almost impossible to police. When we start creating the rules and regulations to make sure there isn't fraud in home health care, there will be quite a substantial bureaucracy.

Some of the things I have learned:

One, you have to involve the doctors in the process if you want to move the health care system. Whether it means educating them better in the medical schools, or making changes in the way they deal with their patients and hospitals, we must be realistic about getting them involved in this process.

Two, the federal government has to be more realistic about what its obvious responsibilities are. In New York City, when I was secretary, the Catholic bishops came to see me to tell me that their parish census had estimated that there were 900,000 undocumented aliens in the city. When Brooklyn Jewish Hospital almost closed, it was not because it wasn't getting Medicaid or Medicare or any other payment; it was because more than half of its patient population was undocumented aliens. There is one part of our system responsible for those people and that is the national government. If the federal government cannot keep them out of this country, it must pick up the tab for their health care.

Three, if Medicaid does not pay for poor people, private health insurance premiums are going to go up because hospitals are going to have to take care of a greater portion of poor people. If those hospitals refuse, the burden will fall on public hospitals funded by the most regressive and controversial source of tax revenue—property taxes—until those hospitals are forced to close their doors in the wake of local taxpayer revolt. Then it will be up to the states again. To the extent states do not do it, the federal government will have to do it. And so on and so forth—a vicious cycle of backdoor health coverage that demeans both the poor and our nation.

And last, I think we know a lot more about what to do about the health care of our poor than some of the pessimistic discussion indicates. I think the problem is not what to do; the problem is whether we can muster the political will to do it. We are the richest country in the history of the world; how can we justify having a health care system that doesn't provide health care for all our people? It is not that doctors don't know how to care for them, or that there are not enough hospital beds to put them in, or that we do not know the medical procedures to help them. It is just that we haven't attended to the problem with the concentration we should have.

6. Response

James H. Sammons

It is hard to argue or to find fault with what Mr. Califano has just said, but there are some things that might bear the light of more discussion. From our perspective there is waste in the system. There is waste because it is a difficult system to administer. There is waste because some of the eligibility requirements are ridiculous. Some are ridiculously high, and others are ridiculously low. There is waste because the system was not designed to save. My preference with Medicaid would be to scrap the whole thing and start over.

There must be some way of making it more efficient without having the federal government take it over with uniform eligibility standards and uniform benefits. If that should happen we might wind up, as did the state of New York at one point, with 50 percent of the population eligible for Medicaid.

For eight years we at the American Medical Association proposed the federalization of Medicaid because of the terrible inconsistencies in the program. Our definition of federalization was somewhat different from the one that the Reagan administration is using. It was also somewhat different from the one that Mr. Califano has just used.

We were pleased with the Reagan administration's concept of block grants and return of the Medicaid system to the states, letting them take over their own policing mechanisms and set their own standards of eligibility. I am concerned by Mr. Reagan's plan to take Medicaid back in 1984. If you have the entire Medicaid program uniformly administered by the Department of Health and Human Services and the entire Medicare program administered by the Department of Health and Human Services, it will be but a small step from there to a total national health program. I am not sure that I agree with the notion that the ills are going to be corrected in a manner that will compensate for the potential dangers in the federalization of Medicaid.

We, too, would share with Mr. Califano the absolute conviction that front-end deductibles and coinsurance, almost irrespective of size, will have a very salutary effect on the program. There is nothing quite like putting the patient through the exercise of participation, even if the participation really doesn't hurt.

Mr. Califano talks about the amount of fraud in the system. I would agree with him it is not anywhere near as extensive as the media have suggested in terms of deliberate fraud by the physician, hospital, and patient. On the other hand, we don't think it ought to be swept under the rug either. When Mr. Califano was secretary, he made some interesting comments about the size of the problem. He may have forgotten these numbers. He said in 1977 that Project

Integrity had turned up 47,000 doctor and pharmacist transactions that needed to be investigated for criminal or civil prosecution. Two years later only about forty had ever been prosecuted. A lot of that is, as Mr. Califano said, because the U.S. attorneys did not want to prosecute. The fraud and abuse problem in the state of Illinois reached such a magnitude that it demanded intervention by the state's attorney and the U.S. attorney. I am convinced that, if you lock some of the thieves up, the rest of them will take their hands out of the cookie jar. We would like to see them incarcerated.

We continue to share Mr. Califano's lack of enthusiasm about national health insurance. But there are gaps in insurance coverage that we have, for years, tried to help resolve. We have made suggestions to the government about filling in those gaps by pooling for the 25 million people who are uninsured. We have recommended changes in the antitrust laws to allow the insurance industry to get in and resolve this problem. When you talk to the federal government about changing antitrust laws, however, it falls on incredibly deaf ears. There are possible solutions to the gap problem and we need to address them, irrespective of what happens to Medicare and Medicaid. I continue to believe that the private sector is the best place to do it. At some time the federal government and the Congress will allow that to happen by changes in the antitrust laws and the insurance statutes.

Mr. Califano says in his paper that he used GMENAC numbers to determine the oversupply of physicians. The American Medical Association does not agree with those numbers or with the conclusions of the GMENAC study. We are seeing some shift in the demographics of the physician population in this country. Whether that is totally due to a recessionary environment, or whether it is in part due to the continuing production of some 15,000 to 16,000 doctors a year doesn't matter. We think that there is clear evidence that it is happening and we do not believe that the shift is going to go the other way.

One of our problems is the almost religious fervor that says 50 percent of all graduates of medical schools must go into primary care. For years, over 50 percent of the graduating seniors in this country have gone, initially at any rate, into primary health care. By giving some sort of slavish obedience to this as a God-given dictate, which it isn't, we are running the risk, it seems to me, of falling into the very trap that we have tried so hard to avoid: determining by fiat the proportionate representation of the various disciplines within the profession.

As long as we are on the manpower problem, two other matters merit discussion. One is the ongoing problem of the American-born foreign medical graduate. What do we do about that American youngster who wants to come home and practice medicine? The other matter concerns the foreign-trained, foreign-born physician coming here from abroad to practice medicine. We need to be more concerned about these two problems than we have been the last couple of years. The overall manpower problem is not going to be resolved until those two issues receive some additional attention.

7. Response

Donald MacNaughton

Mr. Califano chose to open his presentation today by praising the Great Society program and its accomplishments. He pointed out that it had two purposes, the primary one economic. In my opinion the worst economic decision of modern times was the 1965 decision to finance the Great Society program and the escalation of the Vietnam War at the same time without increasing taxes. Much of the inflation that we have been wrestling with ever since dates from that decision.

Let me point out two problems in Mr. Califano's paper. One emerges toward the end, where he describes his desire for a health program administered by the government. He does not describe the program in any specific terms. But then, inconsistently and fortunately for me, he reverses that position.

Another problem arises from his belief that many of the problems of the system will be corrected if we have some kind of wellness or health care program that emphasizes prevention. Much as I agree with him on that score, I don't follow the reasoning that says this would reduce future hospitalization or medical care. I don't know of any significant data that would bear that out. I know of one study that argued that if you don't smoke and if you don't drink too much and if you eat breakfast and a couple of other things like that, you will live eleven years longer if you are a man and eight years longer if you are a woman. Assuming that the study is true, the problem is that, if people do live eleven and eight years longer, their health care will cost more than if they don't. The best way to reduce the cost of your health care is not to keep you alive eleven years longer, but to see that you die eleven years sooner.

Our earlier discussion about what the cost of health care should be is the place where Mr. Califano's paper should have started. You cannot make a very thorough or useful analysis of whether costs are too high unless you have an idea of what they ought to be. Nobody really knows what percentage of the GNP should be devoted to health care. Should it hover around 10 percent as now, or should it be 5 percent or 25 percent? I don't know, and I think none of us really knows. One of the reasons we don't know is that the answer probably would be different for different ages, for different financial circumstances, and for different life-styles. All those things ought to be taken into consideration before we mandate any caps on the percentage of the Gross National Product that should be devoted to health care.

Even more important is the fact that the cost of health care is going to go up no matter what anyone does. One reason is that the scientific and technological revolution, which has been brought about through the genius of people in the medical world, is not about to stop. I don't think we are through performing miracles. The second reason is that the population is aging, and the older it gets the more medical care it will need. The $245 billion that was spent in 1981 will approach $800 billion in 1990. Whether that specific figure is correct or not, the important thing for analysts to consider is that the cost of health care is still going to go up. Rather than dwelling on that fact, we should be dwelling on how that cost should be shared and who in our society should make that decision. How can we best see to it that this cost, which already shows evidence of getting out of hand, is kept in hand while the need for medical care in this country increases?

There are two things that social planners consider relevant. One is inflation, and the other is an increase in the country's productivity. If we were able to get our inflation rate down to somewhere between 3 and 5 percent and if we were able to increase the nation's productivity to the rate we achieved in the fifties and early sixties, the problem that we are now wrestling with would completely disappear, even though the cost of medical care will rise dramatically in the next decade.

I think we should encourage with incentives the development of new types of health care delivery ideas, and I think we are doing that. The HMO movement, which Mr. Califano did a great deal to promote during his period as secretary, is a shining example of that philosophy, and it holds considerable promise. But the biggest impediment to control of health care costs is first day coverage. The best idea of all would be to reduce first day coverage.

I also think it would be wise if we imposed a means test for Medicare. I certainly would not mix Medicaid and Medicare unless there were a means test for Medicare because one is a welfare program and the other is not. We should not mix them unless Medicare becomes a welfare program, and I hope that doesn't happen.

I think, too, we would be better off if we reduced, and wherever possible eliminated, regulations and administrative costs. Where regulations have been done away with, instead of the dire consequences that were predicted, things have eased themselves along to new paths which hold more promise than the old paths we were on.

Somehow or other we must also attack the malpractice problem that is so prevalent in the United States. When I visited a hospital in the United Kingdom, the first impression I got was that the physicians, feeling free from the burden of malpractice suits, seemed to exercise more freedom of judgment in choosing procedures and tests.

The worst idea of Mr. Califano's tenure as secretary was the cap on hospital costs. A cap on hospital costs accomplishes nothing unless it is accompanied by a cap on nurses' salaries, a cap on physicians' fees, a cap on the cost of food, and caps on the cost of pharmaceuticals, hospital equipment, and everything else. Unless you do that, it is impossible to put a cap on hospital costs, unless you assume that hospitals in this country are making too much money. The facts prove the opposite.

There seems to be a feeling that all the poor people of the nation are unfortunates. I agree that those who are unlucky genetically, or unlucky economically, or both, are people who need and should get the help of the rest of society. But should they be treated in the same manner as another large bloc of poor who failed to take advantage of opportunities that came their way? These are the poor who left school instead of staying there, who opted for today's advantages at the sacrifice of tomorrow's. I have the feeling that the two should not be treated the same.

Mr. Califano remarked that he hoped that business would go to the insurance companies and help them reduce the premiums for health insurance policies. I'm not sure whether he meant business should work with insurance companies in that direction, or whether he meant that the premiums are too high and that business really ought to do something about it. If the latter, he should recognize the fact that most of the insurance industry is, and has been for a long time now, making up severe losses in the health insurance business with profits from their life insurance products.

8. Response

Paul Ellwood, Jr.

Mr. Califano seems to hope that an aroused and awakened private sector can help resolve some of the problems associated with providing better health to the poor and aged at prices that the public is prepared to accept. As a practical matter, can the private sector improve the situation of the poor and the elderly? After all, most of the health care that these individuals receive is delivered by private doctors and hospitals. Since I am interested in improving private sector performance by modifying the structure and incentives of the health industry, I'd like to ask whether modification of incentives for the private sector could improve the care provided the poor and the elderly. I would suggest that the answer to that question is "Yes" for the elderly, at least the acutely ill elderly, and a more tentative "Yes" for those on Medicaid, particularly those who require long-term care.

Our analysis of HMOs suggests that competition, capitation payment systems, and putting providers at risk do not at the outset produce major innovations in medical care. They don't produce massive health promotion programs. They don't generate any major new technology, such as computerization of diagnoses and treatments. HMOs have produced savings by reducing the excessive utilization characteristic of the present system. The fact that non-HMO settings like the Mayo Clinic can provide good health care with rates of hospitalization much lower than those of the country as a whole further suggests that we probably provide too much hospitalization. The whole system of HMOs is built on that notion and, to some extent, on improving the organization and delivery of ambulatory care.

Are there analogous excesses in the delivery of acute and long-term care services to the poor and the elderly? Given some new incentives can the private sector effect improvements in the performance of that segment of the system?

Let me start with two pieces of data. The first is some experience with chemical dependency in the Twin Cities. We have had an opportunity to observe private doctors providing chemical dependency services to people in HMOs and the same doctors providing chemical dependency services in hospitals to people on Medicare and Medicaid. In HMOs 35 percent of the dollars are spent on inpatient management and 65 percent on outpatient management of chemical dependency. For Medicare and Medicaid, 85 percent of the dollars are spent on inpatient management and 15 percent on outpatient management of chemical dependency. Those figures give you some hope that modification of the incentives could improve the situation.

Another piece of data comes from Rochester, New York, where we compared the number of days that people on Medicare spend in the hospital prior to being discharged and sent home with the number of days they spend in the hospital before being discharged into a skilled nursing facility. In the case of those who are discharged and sent home, the average number of days is thirty-seven. In the case of those being discharged to a skilled nursing facility, the average is 105 days. Can you imagine the rehabilitation services that could be given with the money spent on sixty-eight days of hospitalization?

These and other examples we could all cite indicate that there still is considerable fat in the Medicare and Medicaid programs. By changing incentives and some of the reimbursement categories, I think we could provide health care and independent living services as good as they are now receiving, or better, at reasonable cost and certainly at lower rates of inflation than we are now experiencing.

Six experiments are now going on in nine different treatment institutions which Medicare is capitating for providing health services to people on Medicare. The institutions are Kaiser in Portland; the Fallon Clinic, which is a fee-for-service group practice in Worcester, Massachusetts; the Marshfield Clinic, a rural fee-for-service group practice; Health Central, an HMO in Lansing, Michigan; International Medical Center, an HMO in Miami, Florida; and four Twin Cities HMOs, three staffed by private physicians and one by salaried physicians.

The hospital utilization rates for Medicare beneficiaries are four thousand days per one thousand people in this country, or four days per person per year. In Kaiser Portland, where the Medicare population is somewhat younger than the average, but not so much younger that it would explain these differences, the average number of hospital days per person per year is 1.7. The Marshfield program, which serves people older and sicker than those who live in the community immediately around the clinic, averages 3.0 days per person per year. In the Twin Cities we are running just over 2.0 days per person per year, about half the average rate.

This is proving to be rather attractive to older people, in spite of the fact that it is an experiment, and in spite of the fact that they have to give up wraparound coverage. Our experiment has been going on for nine months, and 5 percent of the people over sixty-five have joined the program during that period of time. In Marshfield, where people do not have to change doctors, about 45 percent of the population over sixty-five has joined the program during the almost two years that it has been operating.

How do these savings get spent? In return for a premium of about $15 a month Kaiser Portland has offered people on Medicare its most elaborate set of benefits: 365 days of hospitalization, all physician visits without cost, free eyeglasses, free hearing aids, total dental care including fillings and prostheses, and elimination of the problems that are associated with Medicare.

We have also seen some new programs which are beginning to provide something between acute care and long-term care. As these organizations have sought to get people home earlier from the hospital, they have approached nursing homes about keeping people for three or four or five days for physical therapy before they go home. Nursing homes are not set up to do that sort of thing. They are set up to warehouse people for an extended period of time, and not to teach people or to help people live more independently.

A particularly interesting question is whether we can capitate long-term care. Is it possible to take this very difficult population and pay a fixed number of dollars per month for them and realize a lower rate of nursing home use, or savings, or an improvement in the health status or the life-style of these individuals? The most interesting experiment of this type is a program called ONLOK in the Chinese section of San Francisco. The project receives approximately $1,000 per person each month for people who are classified as needing skilled nursing care through a nursing home. Instead, they are living in their own homes or in minimum care facilities. The average per capita cost for Medi-Cal, not including Medicare supplementation, is around $1500 a month, so ONLOK is effecting a one-third saving and the participants are living in more desirable environments.

There are three problems in doing this. The first problem is mixing private and public payment for these kinds of services. There seems to be pretty general agreement that the practice of parents passing on their fortunes to their children and going onto Medicaid is not desirable. I think the uncertainty that so many elderly people feel about the possibility that they will end up in long-term care calls for some new mode of paying for that. Dr. Reinhardt mentioned the notion of long-term care insurance or credits. There was a recent article in *The New England Journal of Medicine* that suggested that such credits be transferable to children in case their parents do not use them. Reverse annuity mortgages are another way of financing long-term care.

The second and perhaps most difficult problem is arriving at a suitable capitation rate. This is true of Medicare and even more true of a program combining Medicare and Medicaid. It is quite clear that in order to capitate Medicare we have to be able to classify people on the basis of their health status in addition to their place of residence, their age and their sex, which is the traditional way of determining capitation rates. When you capitate for long-term care, you have to take into account the homes they live in and whether there is a spouse or some individual with whom they live who can help to take care of them. It becomes a monumental job to determine just how much money is appropriate per month or per year.

The third problem that needs to be resolved is how to deal with the ability of providers to frustrate the intent of change strategies introduced in gradual and piecemeal fashion. For example, hospital utilization has declined in the Twin Cities. With 500,000 people having joined these HMOs in four years, there isn't the demand for hospital services that there used to be. The hospitals had to come up with some way to fill their beds; recent legislation requiring health insurance policies to include twenty-eight days of inpatient mental health coverage helped them out. The average length of stay for mental health in the Twin Cities right now is 27.4 days.

I had hoped that physicians adopting a new set of medical practices in their HMO business would allow that same set of practices to carry over to the rest of their activities. That doesn't appear to happen. In the Twin Cities, 80 percent of the private doctors are in HMOs. Comparing lengths of stay, we find that they hospitalize HMO members for shorter periods than nonmembers. The average length of stay for HMO members hospitalized for perinatal conditions is 39 percent of the average stay for nonmembers. For congenital anomalies, it is 41 percent. For malignancies, it is 63 percent. For benign tumors, it is 91 percent. For pregnancy, it is 100 percent, because pregnancies are managed the same way in both systems. Overall, however, the length of stay for HMO members is about 62 percent of the average stay for nonmembers—same doctors, same hospitals, and same community.

I would like to close with a question to Mr. Califano. In view of recent news reports that the Reagan administration has apparently decided not to push the competitive approach, at least as far as private health insurance and taxes are concerned, is this administration likely to treat the health system as different from the rest of the economy, as an industry that should be singled out for regulation when the rest of the economy is to be spared?

Discussion

Dr. David A. Hamburg: I want to comment on some aspects of health promotion. I doubt whether the subject is likely to come up again, and I think it is very important. But I cannot resist saying something first about economic constraints.

We often talk about economic constraints in this country, where we spend well over $1,000 a year per person for health care. Nearly three-quarters of the world's population spends less than five dollars per person per year for health care. I'm not quite sure what we mean when we talk about economic constraints. It seems to me that it is not so much a question of lack of funds as it is a question of the way we use the funds. I cannot help thinking about a fundamental set of points that Walsh McDermott, late professor emeritus of public health and medicine at Cornell, used to make; namely, that there are some disease problems that cannot be improved without improving socioeconomic conditions, yet there are also some diseases that can be dealt with effectively even in the presence of low socioeconomic status. For the latter case, he gave the example of what happened with tuberculosis in our urban areas when we got effective chemotherapy.

Without losing sight of the profound desirability of improving the socioeconomic status of disadvantaged people, health professionals can address ways of improving health in existing circumstances, and, indeed, such improvements can enhance both the effectiveness and the productivity of poor people and thereby improve their life chances in the long run. Wherever we can prevent serious disease, it is certainly important to do so. It is worth focusing on illness among the poor and elderly where we have an effective intervention in hand or can reasonably foresee an effective intervention with research in the visible future. In point of fact, there are some data indicating that poor people actually receive fewer preventive services than more affluent people. The National Ambulatory Medical Care Survey indicated that disadvantaged minorities are less likely to receive such preventive services as blood pressure checks, Pap smear and breast exams. Generally, preventive care is inversely related to socioeconomic status and that is something we have to address.

There are some opportunities for effective interventions that need not be expensive. To a large extent they involve better public education and ways of reaching a wider segment of our society. A case in point is Mr. Califano's smoking initiative, where very little money was actually spent. Among other things, he used his high office to reach a wider segment of the population than had ever been reached on that subject before. I was delighted to see recently a very effective new surgeon general's report for 1982. More public education of that sort is likely to reach a larger share of our population.

Dr. Feldman at the National Center for Health Statistics has in press a paper showing impressive improvement in mortality rates associated with the attainment of higher levels of education. That study shows how prenatal care, particularly early prenatal care, increases with the mother's education.

Another example is the experience of the National High Blood Pressure Education Program, which has significant policy as well as research implications for the socially disadvantaged. It has certain characteristics that tend to overcome the psychosocial forces that so often interfere with the disadvantaged receiving adequate health care services. One is vigorous and systematic early detection. Another is determined follow-up of treated patients by health professionals. Another is an explicit attempt at patient education. Another is group counseling and, in some locations, the use of social functions or existing social networks to reinforce health promoting behavior with respect to hypertension. Still another is clinic hours that are compatible with the work schedules of poor people. Yet another is providing transportation where necessary. Adherence to a therapeutic regimen is very much higher with that kind of systematic effort than it is ordinarily in low-education, low-income groups.

There have also been several points of ingenuity in major projects involving hypertension in the black community. One is the involvement of the black churches as a way of getting to people who otherwise would be outside the intervention net. Another is the Black Health Care Provider Task Force on Hypertension set up in Mr. Califano's time at HEW, which has now become a private-sector venture between the Red Cross and HHS and black health care providers.

In industry there have been some vigorous attempts to deal with cardiovascular risk factors and alcohol. Companies like Johnson & Johnson, Xerox, IBM, and Coors are using the work site for intervention programs, not only for employees but also for their families.

In prenatal and perinatal medicine the Cleveland Metropolitan Hospital showed a 60 percent reduction in perinatal mortality with a program of patient education, nutrition counseling, social service intervention, and special attention to adolescents, with emphasis again on systematic follow-up to make sure that the intervention is pursued.

There are a number of outcome studies showing that early prenatal care and perinatal care can make a big difference in prematurity and low birth weights, which are concentrated in the low socioeconomic population, especially among early adolescent pregnancies. Anything that can be done in a preventive way in the area of pregnancy has the potential not only to relieve a great deal of human suffering but to save lifelong costs of institutional care, of special education, of all the problems associated with retardation and handicapping conditions.

The final point on disease prevention involves early intervention among adolescents, reaching them at a time when they are initially experimenting with health damaging behaviors—with cigarettes, with alcohol, with vehicles, and with their own bodies. We must learn through research how to make more effective preventive interventions at that stage, before such behavior crystallizes in permanent health-damaging patterns. When we think about how to reach these young people, we should think not only about medical care, but also about the schools which have been a virtual wasteland despite their potential. We should also think about the media. The question is whether health professionals and other leaders in the society can influence the media to make a modest redeployment of the existing investment in their work, in order to have more health promoting effects on adolescents and, for that matter, on all the rest of us. I think we can find ways to intervene more effectively so that poor people and old people and rich people can change their health behavior in more health promoting directions.

Dr. Richard Wilbur: Mr. Califano has made several statements that I would like to comment on. The first is that it is the method of payment of physicians that leads to high cost. Dr. Hans Kotchosky recently showed that multi-specialty clinics, whether or not there is prepayment, have very low hospitalization rates, which may be due to the method of practice and particularly to the encouragement of outpatient procedures.

The implication that the high cost of hospitalization is due to high technology ignores what hospitals pay for. The high cost of hospitals is hotels. Keeping a patient in bed for a day costs a lot of money. Use of high technology outside of the hospital, particularly procedures that can be supervised so that there is no waste or fraud, would probably lower the cost of health care more than tinkering with methods of payment.

Second, I would question the statement that by having physical examinations we can prevent disease. So far as I know, there are no data to support that position. I believe that physical examinations are cost ineffective. You may recall that when the British system was set up forty years ago, there was a promise that the cost, although high, would stay very steady because diseases would be picked up early since patients would come in early. I don't think I need elaborate on the errors in that theory.

Mr. Califano also says that one of our great problems is the maldistribution of physicians by specialty: there are too many in specialties and too few in primary care. When patients are depressed, is it really less expensive to have them see family physicians or psychiatrists, who are trained and usually can take care of the problem more rapidly? I would say the same of many of the diseases seen by dermatologists, particularly skin cancers: going to a specialist more rapidly is probably more cost effective. I should like to see the figures that lie behind the belief that we can lower the overall costs by increasing the number of primary care physicians.

Finally, I would mention the cost of treating illegal aliens in New York hospitals. One reason our health care statistics don't look good is because of the high percentage of aliens who bring in diseases such as tuberculosis that are not seen in our indigenous population. I really question whether tinkering with the health care system is going to take care of the fact that illegal aliens are expensive to take care of. Would it not be better for us to decide whether or not these people are here illegally and either take them into the system or kick them out of the country?

Mr. Califano: Let me just take one second to clarify my position on government involvement in health insurance. I believe that the government should mandate that every employer provide every employee a minimum package of health care benefits. Let the employers go get those benefits in any way they want: provide them themselves, get a government insurance company, or whatever. Make it like the minimum wage, and the bureaucracy will be much smaller than under any other system. For small employers or people who cannot afford that kind of insurance, I would have a government corporation provide it at the going rate for group policies for the large corporations. Lastly, I think we have to pay for poor people and the way to do that is in a common pool, like a city pool, a state pool, or a federal pool. We also have to pay for the old people through Medicare. I would require copayments, but only for those people who can afford them.

With respect to costs, I think that Mr. McNaughton assumes that getting inflation down will necessarily get health care costs down. With a generally inflationary economy, we could perhaps bring costs down some, but they have incessantly run higher than the consumer price index.

The point of cost containment is not that hospitals are making too much money. The point of cost containment is that there is nothing that resembles or will resemble competition in the hospital situation. The reimbursement is essentially cost plus fee-for-service, and there is little incentive to be efficient. There is no relationship of a direct nature between a patient and a hospital, as there is between a buyer and seller. I don't pick the hospital I go to. My family physician sends me to a doctor who picks the hospital. I don't pick the tests I undergo. The people who pick the tests and do them aren't paying for them and, as we all know, I'm not paying for them either. My insurance company is, or Medicare, or Medicaid, or the Blues. Fifty years ago 94 percent of the health care bills were paid personally, and now it's exactly the reverse, as far as hospital bills are concerned.

So, I don't think the system works, and I know nothing short of controls to take care of it until the method of reimbursement is changed. Cost-control legislation has never been proposed as a permanent idea. I don't think when Senator Dole says he wants to look at the matter again, and when the Reagan administration is obviously going to cap hospital costs either by law or regulation, that they view controls as a permanent solution. Until we can change the reimbursement system, people are going to go where the money is.

On physician maldistribution I will just rest on the GMENAC report. I would add just one thing: It is quite clear from studies we did at HEW that the more surgeons you have, the more surgery you have; the more specialists you have, the more specialized care you have. I know Washington has its own mental health problems, but it also has the highest concentration of psychiatrists in the country. The fact that they are the best paid psychiatrists is not unrelated to the fact that the federal government picks up 80 percent of the cost of psychiatric analytic services. Psychiatrists, like hospitals, like doctors, like human beings everywhere, go where the money is.

I think long-term care is a massive problem. We certainly didn't deal with it in the Carter Administration because the numbers are frightening.

I don't think there is a tremendous amount of difference between Medicare and welfare. Millions of people on Medicare are also on Medicaid for their nursing home bills. I think those programs have to be consolidated ultimately.

As far as poor people are concerned, I think we have to remember that they are not a static population. Most of them work, and a good proportion of them work full-time but just don't make enough money to pay all their bills. Our studies indicated that about 20 or 30 percent of the poor people change every year. They move out of poverty one year, and a lot of them slip back in again.

And last, on prevention, I'll close with an anecdote about how important I think prevention is for poor people, not only for their health but also for their opportunities in society. In 1978 I went to the South Bronx and spent half a day at an elementary school there. Every kid in that school was on welfare, and most of their mothers were under twenty.

At the end of the day I sat down with the principal and I said, "What would you do if you had some more money?"

He said, "How much money?"

I said, "I don't know, you tell me!"

He said, "$20,000?"

And I said, "Yes, $20,000. What would you do with it if I gave it to you?"

He said, "I'd hire a nurse!"

And I said, "Why?" It surprised me.

He said, "Because most of the kids here come with learning problems, eye problems, physical problems that they get because their mothers don't get any prenatal care at all. They don't know what to feed them, and they don't know what to do with them before they get to school. In this neighborhood, we know when a girl is pregnant. I'd use that nurse to take care of these kids and their mothers before the kids get to school!"

I think it is important to provide substantial preventive services to the poor that will help a lot of them overcome their problems over the long haul.

Session III

9. Medicare Reconsidered

Karen Davis

For fifteen years the Medicare program has operated with relatively little controversy—steadily paying the health care bills of millions of elderly and disabled Americans. It has won widespread support by relieving the financial burden of health care on the elderly and their families and by ensuring access to hospital and physician services for many of the nation's most vulnerable and critically ill citizens.

Despite its noncontroversial past, Medicare is likely to come under increasing scrutiny in the years ahead. The program will spend almost $50 billion in the 1982 fiscal year, up 17 percent over the previous year.[1] It is a major item in the federal budget, accounting for one out of every fifteen dollars spent by the federal government. As the executive branch and the Congress grapple with alternatives for trimming governmental expenditures, no program will be immune from review—not even the "safety net" Medicare program.[2]

Experience under Medicare

Medicare covers persons age sixty-five and over who receive Social Security or Railroad Retirement cash benefits,[3] about 95 percent of all elderly persons. Beginning in July 1973, Medicare coverage was also extended to individuals permanently and totally disabled for two years or more and to persons with end-stage renal disease.

Medicare consists of two parts: Part A covers hospital, nursing home, and home health services; Part B covers physician services, outpatient hospital services, home health services, and limited other ambulatory services. The program does not cover prescription drugs, dental care, routine eye examinations, eyeglasses, hearing aids, preventive services, or long-term institutional services. Coverage under Part A is extended to all eligible persons; those covered under Part A may voluntarily enroll in Part B coverage by paying a premium. Part A is financed by a payroll tax on employers and employees; Part B is financed by general revenues and premium contributions.

Part A covers inpatient hospital care for ninety days in a spell of illness (a new spell of illness begins when the beneficiary has not been in a hospital or nursing home for sixty continuous days), and for extra days drawn from a sixty-day lifetime reserve. The beneficiary pays a first-day deductible indexed to the cost of hospital care: $260 in 1982, up from $40 in 1966. In addition the beneficiary pays one-fourth of this deductible for the sixty-first to ninetieth day of care, and one-half of this deductible for each day of the lifetime reserve used.

Table 9.1. Trends in Medicare enrollees, reimbursement, and reimbursement per enrollee, 1967–79

	Medicare enrollees (in millions)	Medicare reimbursement (in billions)	Medicare reimbursement per enrollee
1967	19.5	$ 4.5	$ 233
1968	19.8	5.7	287
1969	20.1	6.6	328
1970	20.5	7.1	346
1971	20.9	7.9	376
1972	21.3	8.6	405
1973	23.5	9.6	407
1974	24.2	12.4	513
1975	25.0	15.6	625
1976	25.7	18.4	718
1977	26.5	21.8	823
1978	27.2	24.9	918
1979	27.9	29.3	1,053

Source: Calculated from U.S. Department of Health and Human Services, Health Care Financing Administration, *Medicare and Medicaid Data Book, 1981* (Baltimore: Department of Health and Human Services, Health Care Financing Administration, Office of Research and Demonstrations, 1982), tables 2.1 and 2.6, pp. 13, 20.

The premium for Part B as of July 1981 was $11 per month, up from $3 in July 1966. The beneficiary is responsible for the first $75 of Part B services, 20 percent of all allowable charges after the $75 deductible is met, and any excess of charges actually made by physicians over and above charges the Medicare program sets as allowable. Physicians charge at the Medicare rate on about half of Medicare claims.[4]

States may buy Medicare coverage for the elderly on Medicaid, and most choose to do so. States pay the premium and beneficiary cost sharing under Medicare (with the federal government sharing in the cost at the normal Medicaid federal financial participation rate).

Expenditures: Trends and Distribution among the Elderly

Medicare expenditures have risen rapidly throughout the last fifteen years.[5] Reimbursement for services under Medicare increased from $4.5 billion in 1967, the first full year of the program, to $29.3 billion in 1979. Enrollees over this period increased from 19.5 million elderly in 1967 to 27.9 million elderly and disabled individuals in 1979. The major increase in enrollment occurred in 1973 with the addition of the disabled to the program. By 1979 almost three million Medicare enrollees were covered because of disability, including 20,000 disabled with end-stage renal disease. (See table 9.1.)

Annual rates of increase in payments for services were particularly marked during three periods: the first two years, as the program was implemented; in 1974, as the disabled began receiving services; and in 1975–77, as the removal

Table 9.2. Annual percentage increase in Medicare enrollees, reimbursement, and reimbursement per enrollee, 1968-79

Year	Medicare enrollees	Medicare reimbursement	Medicare reimbursement per enrollee
1968	1.5%	25.2%	23.2%
1969	1.5	15.9	14.3
1970	1.8	7.5	5.5
1971	2.1	10.8	8.6
1972	2.0	9.9	7.7
1973	10.4	10.9	0.5
1974	2.8	30.2	26.0
1975	3.1	24.9	21.8
1976	2.8	18.2	14.9
1977	3.1	18.2	14.6
1978	2.7	14.5	11.5
1979	2.6	17.6	14.7

Note: For base year 1967, Medicare enrollees were 19.5 million; Medicare reimbursement was $4.5 billion; and Medicare reimbursement per enrollee was $233. See table 9.1.
Source: See table 9.1.

Table 9.3. Future projected trends in Medicare budget outlays, 1980-85

Fiscal year	Outlays (billions of $)			Medicare as a percentage of	
	Medicare (current law)	Federal health	Federal budget	Federal health outlays	Federal budget outlays
1980 actual	$35.0	$58.2	$579.6	60.1%	6.0%
1981 actual	42.5	66.0	657.2	64.4	6.3
1982 projected	49.8	73.4	725.3	67.8	6.9
1983 projected	57.1	78.1	757.6	73.1	7.5
1984 projected	65.4	84.9	805.9	77.0	8.1
1985 projected	75.1	93.5	868.5	80.3	8.6

Source: Office of Management and Budget, *Budget of the United States Government, FY 1983* (Washington, D.C.: U.S. Government Printing Office, 1982), tables on pages M-5, 5-130. See also, Office of Management and Budget, *Budget of the United States Government, FY 1982* (Washington, D.C.: U.S. Government Printing Office, 1981), pages M-3, 234, 235.

of wage and price controls under the Economic Stabilization Program resulted in a major surge in health care costs nationwide (see table 9.2).[6] On average, however, Medicare payments per enrollee have increased more markedly than health care expenditures per capita, with reimbursements per enrollee increasing from $233 in 1967 to $1,053 in 1979.

Future projections indicate that no slowdown in expenditure growth is anticipated. Medicare budgetary outlays are projected to increase from $35 billion in FY 1980 to $50 billion in FY 1982 to $75 billion in FY 1985 (see table 9.3). These increases projected under the current Medicare law are substantial, even

Table 9.4. Percentage distribution of Medicare expenditures by type of service

Type of service	Percentage distribution					
	1970		1975		1980	
Hospital	68.0	($5.1)	71.2	($11.6)	71.7	($26.3)
Physician	21.3	(1.6)	20.2	(3.3)	21.0	(7.7)
Nursing home	4.0	(0.3)	1.8	(0.3)	1.1	(0.4)
Other services	1.3	(0.1)	1.8	(0.3)	3.3	(1.2)
Administrative expenses	5.3	(0.4)	4.3	(0.7)	3.0	(1.1)
Total	100.0	($7.5)	100.0	($16.2)	100.0	($36.7)

Note: Figures in parentheses are Medicare expenditures (billions of $) for the adjacent percentages.
Source: Robert M. Gibson and Daniel R. Waldo, "National Health Expenditures, 1980," *Health Care Financing Review*, 3, no. 1 (September 1981): 42, 45, 46.

when viewed in relation to other federal budgetary expenditures. If the program continues unchanged, Medicare will account for 80 percent of the president's projected health outlays in FY 1985, up from 60 percent in 1980, and increase from 6.0 percent of total federal budgetary outlays in 1980 to 8.6 percent in 1985.[7] The most recent acceleration in Medicare expenditures again reflects an explosion in health care costs, especially in the hospital sector.[8]

Medicare expenditures go primarily for hospital and physician services. In 1980 72 percent of Medicare expenditures went for hospital care, a little over one-fifth of all expenditures were paid for physicians' services, only one percent of payments supported nursing home care, and administrative expenses represented 3 percent of total expenditures (see table 9.4). Given the predominance of hospital services in Medicare expenditures, it is not surprising that total program expenditures are sensitive to national trends in hospital costs.

These averages for the program as a whole, however, mask the extreme variability among the elderly and disabled in their need for and use of health care services. Medicare enrollees are a far from homogeneous population. Many of the elderly are healthy and rarely use health care services.[9] Others have multiple chronic problems requiring extensive care and treatment. Some 77 percent of the elderly have annual Medicare reimbursements of less than $500 and account for 5.4 percent of all Medicare reimbursements for the elderly. At the other extreme, 8.8 percent of the elderly have average annual Medicare payments of over $3,000 and account for 70 percent of all Medicare expenditures. Or looking at it another way, 8.8 percent of the elderly have average Medicare payments of $7,011, while at the opposite extreme, 36.8 percent of the elderly have average Medicare payments of $129 annually, and 39.8 percent of elderly Medicare enrollees have no payments.

As startling as these figures are, they are not unrepresentative of the distribution of expenditures for younger age groups. The Congressional Budget Office estimates that approximately 85 percent of the under 65 population either incurs no health care expenditures during the year or has expenditures under $500.[10] But 3.5 percent of the under age 65 population accounts for 50 percent of all health expenditures of the nonaged, with average bills in excess of $2,500. Skewing of health expenditures would appear to be a reflection of patterns of illness that affect the entire population rather than a reflection of the Medicare program.

A new study has found that Medicare pays the medical bills of many of those who die.[11] About 65 percent of those who died in 1965 were Medicare enrollees. Not surprisingly, those who died during the year were more likely to have required health care services than those who survived. As a result, Medicare spent $3,351 per person dying in 1976 during the last twelve months of life compared with $509 per survivor. Decedents represented 6.4 percent of enrollees, and Medicare expenditures in the last twelve months of life accounted for 31 percent of Medicare payments. Decedents were much more likely to be hospitalized; 75 percent of decedents and 19 percent of survivors had hospital stays in a twelve-month period. Average stays of decedents were slightly longer, 13.8 days compared with 10.4 days. Since 75 percent of all deaths of persons over age sixty-five are for heart disease, cancer, and cerebrovascular diseases, a hospital episode in the last twelve months of life is probably to be expected.[12]

These studies and recent data provide more insight into the nature of Medicare expenditures than was previously available from aggregate data. They suggest that Medicare is primarily a program for those with serious health care problems. While it is undoubtedly important for those with routine medical problems, the bulk of all expenditures are concentrated on a minority of the elderly faced with life-threatening conditions.

Medicare's Accomplishments

Financial burden of health care expenditures. Much of the impetus for the Medicare program came from the desire to lighten the burden of heavy medical expenses for the aged. The 1963 Social Security survey of the aged documented that about half of them had no private health insurance.[13] As individuals retired, they lost their employer group insurance. Companies were reluctant to write individual comprehensive policies for the elderly for fear they would insure an excessive number of poor risks. Thus, remedying the failure of the private market to provide adequate health insurance at affordable cost was the chief goal of the Medicare program. Medicare has clearly been highly successful in meeting this goal. Without Medicare, medical bills for the 10 to 20 percent of the elderly with serious health problems would be a devastating financial burden on the elderly and their families.

While Medicare has afforded considerable financial protection for the elderly for the services it covers, restrictions on its benefit package mean that the elderly continue to pay extensive medical bills. Medicare picks up 44 percent of the personal health expenditures of the elderly. Other public programs, primarily Medicaid, contribute another 19 percent. The remaining 37 percent, or an aver-

Table 9.5. Personal health expenditures per person age 65 and over by type of service and source of payment, 1978

	Personal health expenditures per person age 65 and over	Distribution by source of payment			
		Medicare	Other Public	Private	Total
Hospital	869	74.6	12.9	12.5	100.0
Physician	366	55.6	3.8	40.6	100.0
Nursing home	518	3.0	43.2	53.8	100.0
Drugs	133	—	15.6	84.4	100.0
Dental	57	—	3.2	96.8	100.0
Other	84	31.3	16.4	52.3	100.0
Total	$2,026	44.1	19.1	36.8	100.0

Source: Charles R. Foster, "Differences by Age Groups in Health Care Spending," *Health Care Financing Review*, 1, no. 4 (Spring 1980): 81.

age of $746 per elderly person in 1978, is paid directly by the elderly or through private health insurance. (See table 9.5.)

Coverage varies a great deal by type of service. Medicare pays 75 percent of the elderly's hospital bills, and other public programs pay 13 percent, leaving only 12 percent to be paid by the elderly. Medicare pays 56 percent of physician expenditures, with the elderly responsible for 41 percent. Medicare pays only 3 percent of nursing home expenditures, although Medicaid and other public programs pay 43 percent. Still, nursing home care is a major financial burden on the elderly and their families, with 54 percent of nursing home expenditures paid privately. Medicare pays none of the $190 spent per elderly person on drugs and dental services.

Despite Medicare, the elderly pay considerably more out-of-pocket for health care than the nonelderly. In 1978 the average private payment for health expenditures for the nonelderly was $426, compared with $746 for the elderly.[14] In 1975, 8 percent of the elderly had out-of-pocket health expenses of $1,000 or more, compared with 3 percent of the nonelderly population.[15] Out-of-pocket expenses are particularly burdensome for the poor or nearly poor who are elderly. In 1970 aged families with incomes near the poverty level spent 13 percent of their income on medical expenditures, though younger families with low incomes averaged only 7 percent, and younger families with incomes above the near-poverty level paid 4 percent.[16]

Access to care. While the primary objective of Medicare was to protect the aged against the possibility of large medical outlays, the program was also concerned to eliminate financial barriers that discourage the elderly from seeking medical care.

Medicare did result in a major increase in utilization of hospital services by the elderly. Hospital admission rates climbed steeply in the first years of the program, leveled off during the period 1969–71, and climbed steadily since that time. Since 1971 lengths of hospital stay have shortened, so that total days of hospital care per elderly person have been relatively stable since 1971.

Studies of the impact of Medicare on utilization of services found that the major initial impact of the program was on subgroups in the elderly population traditionally identified as most in need of care—individuals living alone with low incomes, minorities, residents of the South and nonmetropolitan areas.[17]

Certain types of surgical procedures also increased dramatically with the introduction of the program. Cataract operations doubled between 1965 and 1975, and arthroplasty nearly tripled, leading some analysts to conclude that the quality of life for the aged improved as a result of Medicare.[18]

Medicare does not appear to have dramatically changed ambulatory physician services received by the elderly. Physician visits per elderly person averaged 6.7 visits per person in 1964 and 6.6 visits per person in 1980.[19] However, the elderly did receive increasing amounts of in-hospital physician services, related to the increasing hospitalization and surgery. Between 1971 and 1977 physicians' charges for services rendered in the inpatient hospital setting increased by 125 percent, compared with a 92 percent increase in physician charges for services rendered to ambulatory patients.[20]

Health status. While Medicare's objectives were concerned primarily with the financial burden of health care and assuring access to care, studies confirm that the health of the elderly improved after the introduction of Medicare. Bernard Friedman, for example, found that the elderly had fewer days of restricted activity and that this decline was inversely related to the level of personal health care expenditures by the aged.[21] His study revealed that the mortality rates of aged males in 1969 were lower than might have been predicted from previous experience.

More recent data underscore the sharp decline in mortality among the aged since the introduction of Medicare. During the period from 1955 to 1967 mortality rates of aged males increased slightly, while death rates for aged females declined at an annual rate of one percent. But in the 1968–1977 Medicare period, death rates for both elderly men and women took a sharp downward turn. Death rates for elderly males declined at an annual rate of 1.5 percent and for women at an annual rate of 2.3 percent.[22]

These rates of decline are much more dramatic than those experienced by the elderly in Canada and European countries over this period. In table 9.6, the average annual decline in death rates for elderly men during 1968 to 1977 was 0.6 percent in Canada and European countries, compared with 1.5 percent in the U.S. Death rates of elderly women declined 1.7 percent in Canada and European countries compared with 2.3 percent in the U.S.

A careful analysis of mortality experience of the elderly in the U.S. by Rosenwaike et al. concludes that the steep downward trend in mortality is a real phenomenon rather than a statistical artifact.[23] The study notes the particularly marked decline for the population over age eighty-five, and the marked declines

Table 9.6. Average annual percentage change in age-adjusted death rates for persons 65 years of age and over (selected countries)

Country	1955–67	1968–77
Males age 65 and over		
United States	0.2%	–1.5%
Canada	–0.4	–0.8
England and Wales	–0.3	–1.0
France	–1.0	–0.3
German Federal Republic	–0.1	–1.2
Netherlands	0.1	–0.2
Sweden	–0.1	–0.1
Average, other than U.S.	–0.3	–0.6
Females age 65 and over		
United States	–1.0	–2.3
Canada	–1.6	–1.9
England and Wales	–0.9	–1.0
France	–1.8	–1.2
German Federal Republic	–1.7	–2.1
Netherlands	–1.7	–2.3
Sweden	–1.6	–1.9
Average, other than U.S.	–1.6	–1.7

Source: U.S. Department of Health and Human Services, National Center for Health Statistics, *Health, United States, 1981* (Hyattsville, Md., 1981), p. 30.

in deaths with an underlying cause assigned to cardiovascular conditions and to cerebrovascular diseases. Improved medical care treatment for coronary heart disease and stroke is pointed to as an important contributor to this decline.

Drake also attributes the marked decline in mortality to the Medicare program.[24] He notes that one-third of the total increased longevity achieved by a sixty-five year-old in the first seventy-five years of this century occurred in the ten years from 1965 to 1975. Yet he points out that despite this decline, there has been no increase in disability among those surviving, and that almost 70 percent of the elderly rate their health as good or excellent.

While definitive conclusions are difficult to reach and multiple factors have undoubtedly contributed to this significant improvement in the health of the elderly, it would appear that Medicare has had a largely unanticipated impact on the health and life-expectancy of the elderly.

Policy Options

While the Medicare program has enjoyed widespread support, pressures on the executive branch and the Congress to alter the program to curb rising expenditures will increase. These pressures have less to do with the performance of the Medicare program than with the size of the federal budget deficit. The Omnibus Reconciliation Act passed by the Congress in 1981 cut Medicare expenditures for FY 1983 by $1.0 billion.[25] The administration has proposed an additional $3.0 billion savings in the 1982 Medicare budget for FY 1983 and has indicated its intention to submit future legislation to cut Medicare by $24.6 billion between FY 1984 and FY 1987. The legislative and administrative changes enacted in 1981, the changes proposed in 1982, and the future legislation the administration intends to propose would yield Medicare savings of $48.4 billion from FY 1983 to FY 1987.[26] Medicare has slipped out of the safety net.

Administration FY 1983 Medicare Proposals

The administration has proposed a series of immediate measures to reduce federal budgetary outlays for the Medicare program. Together these proposals would add $3.0 billion in FY 1983 savings to the $1.0 billion enacted by Congress last year. These proposals are of three basic types: those that would increase cost sharing by the elderly for covered services, those that would reduce provider reimbursement levels, and those that would generate additional sources of revenue for the program, or shift costs to other parties (see table 9.7).

Proposals that would increase cost sharing by the elderly have particular drawbacks. Indexing the Part B deductible would add to the already substantial out-of-pocket payments for physician services by the elderly. In 1978, Medicare met only 54 percent of physician expenditures of the elderly (excluding the premium paid by the elderly, the government's contribution is less than 36 percent).[27] The Omnibus Reconciliation bill passed last year increased the deductible under Part B from $60 to $75, further reducing the share of expenditures met by Medicare.[28]

Many of the provider reimbursement proposals would exacerbate this problem. Hospitals would not be permitted to charge patients for lowered Medicare reimbursement, but physicians could and likely would simply increase charges to patients to compensate for lowered reimbursement by Medicare. Thus, the elderly's expenditures on physician services for charges in excess of Medicare allowable charges could be expected to rise substantially under the reimbursement proposals.

The 2 percent across-the-board reduction in Medicare hospital cost reimbursement would do little to control rising costs in the hospital sector, but it could lead to discrimination against elderly patients, it would penalize hospitals with lower costs, it would have a disproportionate impact on hospitals carrying a heavier Medicare patient load, and it would do little to lay the groundwork for a more rational system of hospital reimbursement. Details of a new utilization review system are not spelled out. Repeal of the PSRO program without an effective alternative could well lead to higher costs.

The proposals to tap other sources of revenues for meeting health expenditures of the elderly are a natural outgrowth of the absence of any strategy to

Table 9.7. Major provisions of the three basic proposals for reducing federal outlays for Medicare

Provisions	FY 1983 savings[a] (millions of $)
Increased cost-sharing	
Index the Part B deductible to the consumer price index	$ 65
Institute 5 percent coinsurance for home health services	35
Delay initial eligibility by one month	145
Reduce provider reimbursement	
Cut hospital reimbursement by 2 percent	653
Delay update in physician fee screens from July to October	210
Limit increase in physician prevailing fees to 5 percent	35
Reimburse radiologists and pathologists at 80 percent of reasonable charges	160
Limit outpatient department physician reimbursement	160
Implement a composite rate reimbursement system for end stage renal disease services	130
Employ other reimbursement changes	82
Make use of utilization review, repeal of PSRO program, and other proposals	490
Other revenue sources	
Require federal employees to pay Medicare payroll tax	619
Require employers to cover working aged under employee health insurance plans	306
Total	$3,090

a. Savings quoted in U.S. Department of Health and Human Services budget documents are slightly different.
Source: Office of Management and Budget, *Budget of the U.S. Government, FY 1983, Major Themes and Additional Budget Details* (Washington, D.C.: U.S. Government Printing Office, 1982), pp. 59, 60.

contain rising costs directly. If expenditures for the elderly are going to rise inexorably, each party can be expected to attempt to shift a portion of that cost onto some other party.

For federal employees, the proposal represents a reduction in wages without any commensurate benefits of improved health insurance coverage in old age. If federal employee wages are felt to be too high, they should be cut. If they are felt to be at the right level, but folding them into Medicare is a more rational way to provide for their health insurance coverage in retirement, federal employees should receive a wage hike to compensate for the added tax burden.

Requiring employers to extend employee health insurance coverage to working elderly employees could pose a disincentive for employers to hire or retain older workers. Working elderly could feel a double burden—they have contributed throughout their working lifetime to payroll taxes to pay for Medicare, yet they and their employers would have to pay for private health insurance coverage to replace Medicare benefits. The administrative problems of coordinating employer health insurance coverage with secondary Medicare coverage could also be substantial.

Cost Sharing

One proposal would require the elderly to pay a coinsurance rate on hospital care. Medicare requires beneficiaries to pay a first-day deductible ($260 in 1982 and about $300 in 1983). Coinsurance charges at the rate of 25 percent of the first-day deductible are assessed for each day of hospital care beyond sixty days (50 percent for the lifetime reserve which begins after ninety days). No coinsurance is charged presently for care from the second through the sixtieth day of hospital care.

The Congressional Budget Office has developed one option along this line.[29] Under this plan, beneficiaries would be required to pay 10 percent of the cost of the deductible for the second through the thirty-first days of a hospital stay in each calender year—i.e., about $30 per day in 1983. Medicare would cover all charges in excess of any stay beyond thirty-one days, or of separate stays above thirty-one days in a year, thus improving coverage for participants with unusual hospitalization needs. Enrollees would pay only one $300 deductible, no matter how many times hospitalized in a year. This option implicitly sets a maximum yearly out-of-pocket individual liability for hospital costs of about $1,200 for 1983. Medicaid would continue to pay the coinsurance costs for those elderly and disabled persons enrolled in both programs. Enactment of this proposal would save about $7.4 billion over the period from FY 1983 to FY 1987 according to CBO estimates.[30] The objective of such a proposal would be to reduce the federal budgetary outlay for Medicare and to encourage the elderly to avoid hospitalization or to shorten the length of stay if medically possible.

Several questions could be raised about this proposal. First, how large an economic burden would this proposal place on the elderly? As noted earlier, the elderly spent $745 on health care services in 1978, a sum that is likely to increase to around $1,430 in 1983 under current law. Hospitalized patients could expect to have somewhat higher out-of-pocket payments than the average for all elderly. Therefore, adding coinsurance of $900 could easily run out-of-pocket costs to around $2,500 for the 20 percent of the elderly who are hospitalized each year.[31] In 1980, the median income of the elderly was $4,226;[32] although it is somewhat higher now, the elderly are not a high income group.

A second question is whether this proposal would reduce unnecessary hospital utilization among the elderly. A recent report on a health insurance experiment by the Rand Corporation for the nonelderly population found that cost sharing reduces admission rates to hospitals (although the Rand study did not find any effect of coinsurance on lengths of hospital stay).[33] The Rand study, however, provides no evidence on whether the utilization eliminated is for essential hospital care or for marginal hospital care. Nor is it clear that the results of the Rand study would apply to the elderly population. Another study has found that elderly who do not supplement Medicare with private health insurance have lower utilization of services than those who eliminate cost sharing with supplementary insurance.[34] Again, this study provides no evidence on whether such a reduction in utilization is desirable or harmful.

It is clear that the extensive supplementary health insurance purchased by the elderly would mitigate the effects of coinsurance charged by Medicare. The 1979 Current Population Survey found that 43 percent of the elderly have Medicare coverage only, while the rest have either Medicaid or supplementary private insurance.[35] Medicare only coverage is systematically greater for low-income elderly (i.e., 57 percent with incomes below $2,000 have Medicare only, compared with 20 percent of those with incomes over $15,000). Seventy-three percent of those with Medicare only coverage have incomes under $6,000. Institution of hospital coinsurance would result in higher premiums for those elderly who supplement, but very little change in actual use of hospital services. The main economic impact is going to be on the 43 percent of the elderly, primarily low-income elderly, who do not have supplemental coverage.

Analysis of the economic burden and efficiency results of coinsurance also needs to consider the extreme variability of Medicare expenditures among the elderly. Twelve percent of the elderly have charges in excess of $2,000 per year. Seventy-seven percent of the elderly incur charges of less than $500 per year. It is clear that the $7.4 billion that the federal government would save from this proposal over the period FY 1983 to FY 1987 would be borne primarily by the estimated 3 million elderly each year with charges in excess of $2,000. For those elderly with such large gross charges, little marginal effects on hospital utilization could be expected, in large part because such individuals are sure to exceed the ceiling established under the proposal.

In short, the opportunities for improving efficiency in the use of hospital services are limited under cost-sharing proposals, and the possible economic burden on the elderly is quite substantial. Such proposals would essentially represent a tax on the sickest and least affluent segments of society.

Medicare Vouchers

Another long-term approach to the Medicare program would be to permit or require the elderly to purchase private health insurance or enroll in prepaid health plans with vouchers provided in lieu of Medicare benefits. One such legislative proposal is the Voluntary Medicare Option Act introduced by Congressmen Gradison and Gephardt in October 1981.[36] This bill would establish a voucher program as an optional alternative to the current Medicare program. Beginning in 1984, an amount based on the average per capita cost of Medicare adjusted to reflect differences in disability status, age, sex, and residence would be calculated and increased annually by the medical care component of the consumer price index. Elderly and disabled Medicare beneficiaries could use this amount to purchase private health insurance or enroll in prepaid health plans.[37] Eligible plans would be required to cover those services covered by Medicare and enrollees would be guaranteed a "maximum permissible financial participation amount." If premiums for private plans were less than the Medicare voucher, plans could rebate such amounts to enrollees. At the end of a year, enrollees could return to Medicare if they chose.

The earlier Stockman-Gephardt bill had similar provisions.[38] Major differences were that, once in a private plan, beneficiaries could not return to Medicare; Medicare would be abolished once participation in private plans reached 60 percent; plans would not be required to cover all Medicare benefits; and maximum patient out-of-pocket expenses would initially be set at $2,900 (to be indexed by the GNP price deflator).

Proponents of this approach argue that it will foster competition in the health care market. Elderly individuals would have an incentive to purchase private health insurance with more cost sharing than Medicare, thus giving them an incentive to use services more efficiently. With vouchers, more elderly would have an incentive to join lower cost health maintenance organizations. New organizations providing health care services might be formed to gain Medicare enrollee business. Private health insurance plans would have an incentive to negotiate lower provider reimbursement rates in order to offer private health insurance to the elderly at a lower premium. Private health insurance administration might prove to be more flexible and efficient than Medicare.[39]

The first major concern raised by this proposal is the possibility of adverse risk selection. If a voucher at the average value of Medicare, estimated to be approximately $2,200 in FY 1984, is given to Medicare enrollees to purchase private health insurance, this voucher will provide extremely generous private coverage and cash rebates for 76.6 percent of Medicare enrollees whose Medicare expenditures average $62 per year, but it will be far from adequate for the 8.8 percent whose Medicare expenditures average $7,000 per year. Private plans may try to enroll the healthier population by screening on the basis of medical history or by providing poor service to any high risk elderly who enroll. Whether by design or by chance, private plans with good risks will fare well, while those with poor risks will quickly go out of business. If poor risks remain in Medicare, the total cost of the program could well rise.

Preventing adverse risk selection would require careful calibration of the Medicare voucher amount for the health status of the particular enrollee, and strict regulation of marketing, enrollment, and disenrollment practices. Yet this seems virtually impossible to do, and experience to date provides very little evidence that it can be done successfully.

The second concern is whether private health insurance companies could provide Medicare benefits at the same or lower costs. Two factors suggest that costs would be higher under private plans for the same benefits to the same risk population. First, Medicare pays hospitals and physicians at rates below those paid by private insurance plans. In the case of hospital care, it is estimated that Medicare payments are 17 percent below charges paid by commercial insurance companies.[40] Second, Medicare administrative expenses are quite low, averaging 3 percent of benefit payments.[41] Individual insurance policies, on the other hand, have high administrative expenses including sales commissions, advertising, and other marketing expenses. On average, administrative expenses in such plans run 30 to 50 percent of benefit payments.[42] Hence, private health insurance executives have testified publicly that private carriers could not deliver the same benefits for the premium provided, and have indicated privately that their costs could well run 35 to 40 percent more than Medicare's.[43]

While this approach is billed as an alternative to regulation, in fact it is likely to entail considerable regulation. Experience with the Medi-Gap supplementary insurance program has revealed numerous instances of abuses in the sale of private health insurance policies to the elderly.[44] To prevent these abuses, regulations regarding benefits covered, cost-sharing provisions, exclusions of certain services under certain conditions, exemptions of pre-existing conditions, marketing practices, financial soundness of plans, enrollment and disenrollment procedures, truth in advertising, and so forth are likely to be part and parcel of any such proposal. The approach is not an alternative to regulation, but rather the redirection of regulation from health care providers to health insurers.

The major drawback or virtue of the proposal, depending upon one's viewpoint, is that the voucher might not keep pace with the cost of medical care for the elderly resulting in shifting of the cost to the elderly (or alternatively saving money for the federal government). The specific legislative proposals that have been advanced all index benefits at considerably less than Medicare expenditures can be expected to increase over time. Thus, many of the same considerations regarding the economic burden on the elderly raised by cost-sharing proposals apply to voucher approaches as well.

Prospective Reimbursement and Targeted Utilization Review

Another approach would be to take a fundamental look at the way Medicare pays hospitals and physicians and move to a system of prospective reimbursement with built-in, system-wide cost restraints. In a recent speech to the American Hospital Association, Senator Dole expressed his keen disappointment at the failure of the hospital industry to control hospital costs voluntarily and issued a stern warning that the Congress would not stand by while hospital costs increased at double the general rate of inflation.[45] He indicated that the time is long overdue for a major reform in the method of reimbursement for hospitals, and urged the development of a prospective reimbursement system. He indicated that expansion of the current Medicare 223 limits on hospital reimbursement to cover all hospital costs could provide the basis for the formulation of prospective rates. He also expressed concern with Medicare's high return on equity for proprietary hospitals, and noted that physician reimbursement would not be overlooked in any attempt to reduce Medicare expenditures.

The Congressional Budget Office has developed a first-step proposal in this direction.[46] This option would extend Medicare 223 limits (which currently place a ceiling on maximum cost reimbursement for hospital routine costs) to all hospital costs. CBO estimates that this proposal would save $5 billion between FY 1983 and FY 1987. This proposal involves a reimbursement ceiling of 110 percent of mean costs of similar hospitals, adjusted for diagnostic case mix and area wage rates and other input factor costs. It contains a hold-harmless provision to prevent individual hospitals in the early years from receiving less reimbursement than they had in previous years.

Reimbursement ceilings would give higher cost hospitals an incentive to reduce costs. Hospitals that eliminated unnecessary diagnostic services and treatments and shortened hospital stays would be relative gainers under this approach. This is only an intermediate step on the way to a system in which similar hospitals are paid the same rate for providing care to similar patients. For such an approach to be cost restraining, limits on increases over time would need to be established. To avoid discrimination against Medicare patients, similar restraints would have to be established for Medicaid patients and privately insured patients. A cooperative effort involving governmental payers, hospitals, physicians, insurers, business, and labor will be necessary to work out a reimbursement system that will achieve overall cost restraint and provide incentives for encouraging efficiency in the hospital sector.

Reform of physician reimbursement methods under Medicare is also badly needed. Studies have indicated that the usual, customary, and prevailing charge method used by Medicare encourages physicians to raise charges in order to increase future reimbursement rates.[47] The current system is also inequitable, and leads to widely varying fees for the same service provided by different physicians in the same geographical area, and across geographical areas. Development of uniform fee schedules in given geographical areas, with limits on increases over time linked to agreed-upon goals for overall increases in physician expenditures, needs to be undertaken. To avoid shifting costs to the elderly, physicians participating in Medicare should be required to accept the established fee as payment in full. Medicare beneficiaries should be supplied with information on physicians willing to participate in the program under these conditions.

New approaches to reviewing the necessity of utilization of services under Medicare are also needed. Given the large proportion of Medicare expenditures going for a relatively small fraction of Medicare beneficiaries, special utilization review systems should be established to review claims for these individuals. Economic incentives, which result in serious financial strain or even bankruptcy for these individuals, are obviously of limited utility. Direct review of claims for this population would appear to be a more humane way of attempting to ferret out any unnecessary utilization. Assessment of specialized procedures for this population should also be undertaken, to lay the basis for guidelines for coverage of efficacious procedures.

Long-term Care and Catastrophic Coverage

While most changes proposed for the Medicare program are directed at reducing program expenditures, improved coverage of some services needs to be pursued when resources permit. The most obvious limitation of the Medicare program is the virtual absence of long-term care coverage and catastrophic coverage.

Senator Orrin Hatch has proposed a major expansion of Medicare coverage for home health services.[48] His Community Home Health Services Act would provide funds under the Public Health Service Act for the establishment of home health programs and training professional and paraprofessional home health services personnel. It would extend coverage under Medicare for home health services to homebound individuals in need of homemaker-home health aide services on an intermittent basis, where in the absence of such services the individual would require institutionalization. The bill also amends the tax code to provide tax credits of up to $500 for families caring for a disabled dependent. Maximum credits are available to families with incomes less than $30,000 and phase down to zero for families with incomes of $40,000. The Congressional Budget office estimates the cost of this proposal to be $2.4 billion in the first nine months of the program,[49] which makes it a difficult sort of proposal to move forward in the economic climate of 1982.

Although costly, this bill addresses a very real need. In communities across this country, thousands of elderly individuals live alone but are unable to care for themselves without assistance. Approaches to enable these individuals to live out their lives with dignity, avoiding their most dreaded fear of institutionalization, must be carefully explored.

The administration's recent proposal to federalize the Medicaid program provides an excellent opportunity to re-examine the way in which Medicare and Medicaid cover nursing home care, home health care, and other long-term care services.[50] Federalization would permit an integrated approach to this problem, rather than assigning acute care to the federally-funded Medicare program, and long-term care to the federal-state shared Medicaid program. New thinking and approaches in this area are very much needed.

Finally, Medicare will only completely achieve its goal of providing financial protection against medical bills for the elderly if a reasonable ceiling on maximum out-of-pocket expenses of the elderly is added to the program, and coverage is expanded to include such costly items as prescription drugs. As long as cost sharing is unlimited, elderly individuals will continue to live in fear that their meager resources could be exhausted in the event of a catastrophic illness.

Summary

In the last fifteen years Medicare has established itself as a highly successful program. It has been run well for the most part, has filled a gap in private health insurance coverage existing prior to the program, and has achieved its goals of ensuring access to health care services and reducing the severe financial burden of health care bills for the elderly. Death rates of the elderly have plummeted, and the health of the elderly has improved markedly since it began. Despite this record, rapidly rising costs and the prominent role of the Medicare program in the federal budget are creating pressures for major changes. These proposals need to be carefully evaluated, with a view to retaining the progress that has been made, while we explore ways of improving efficiency and reducing cost.

Those proposals which emphasize economic incentives for the elderly, such as increased cost sharing or Medicare vouchers, would appear to have limited utility. Medicare expenditures are highly skewed. Some elderly are relatively healthy and require little medical attention. Other suffer from multiple problems and make recurring use of the health care system. The vast majority of all Medicare expenditures go for the latter group. To expect these individuals to bear a greater proportion of their medical expenses is unrealistic, given the relatively limited incomes and economic resources of this group.

More promising are attempts to change the incentives for health care providers through major reform of the methods of paying for services. For hospitals, prospective reimbursement methods with built-in cost restraints are the most obvious direction to turn. Methodological advances of the last few years and increasing experience with cost ceilings related to efficiency under Medicare 223 limits underscore the feasibility of moving in this direction now, rather than in the future. A cooperative effort, with negotiation between those providing services and those paying for services, should be at the top of the health policy agenda.

Similar efforts should be undertaken with physicians. The inefficiency, inequity, and inflationary pressures of the current methods of physician reimbursement are well known. Rather than continuing along a course unsatisfactory to all parties, we should chart a course toward a rational system of fees in which all physicians would be paid the same rate for the same service in the same geographical area. Such a system should be developed through negotiations involving physicians and public and private payers of services.

But new approaches to Medicare should not be concerned solely with cost constraint. The size of the very old population is increasing, bringing with it new needs for long-term care. Approaches that would enable more people to live out their lives in the community, without losing their independence, need to be closely examined. Proposals to federalize the Medicaid program afford an excellent opportunity to rethink Medicare and Medicaid provisions for long-term care and to move away from excessive reliance upon long-term institutionalization.

Catastrophic protection for the elderly and expanding Medicare's benefits should also be high priorities, as resources permit. It is clear that many elderly and their families would be ruined financially without Medicare and that the remaining burdens are still heavy for some elderly individuals. Further steps in this direction are clearly warranted.

Improvements in the Medicare program will have to compete with much needed improvements in health financing coverage of the poor, child health assurance, primary care for rural and inner-city areas, prevention, and other health priorities. Even so, Medicare improvements of this kind should form an essential component of any health improvement act designed to assure that all our nation's citizens have a right to the pursuit of health.

Notes

1. Office of Management and Budget, *Budget of the U.S. Government, FY 1983* (Washington, D.C.: U.S. Government Printing Office, 1982).

2. In the FY 1982 budget Medicare was listed as a "safety net" program, along with Social Security, veterans' benefits, and unemployment compensation. They were to be immune from proposed cuts.

3. For more detailed discussion of Medicare eligibility, see Bennett Hirsch, Herbert A. Silverman, and Allen Dobson, *Medicare: Health Insurance for the Aged and Disabled, 1976–1978: Summary-Utilization and Reimbursement by Person* (Baltimore: Health Care Financing Administration, in press).

4. Thomas P. Ferry, Marian Gornick, Marilyn Newton, and Carl Hacherman, "Physicians' Charges Under Medicare: Assignment Rates and Beneficiary Liability," *Health Care Financing Review* (winter 1980).

5. For an in-depth review of the first ten years of the Medicare program, see Karen Davis and Cathy Schoen, *Health and the War on Poverty: A Ten Year Appraisal* (Washington, D.C.: Brookings Institution, 1978).

6. See Stuart Altman, testimony before the U.S. House of Representatives, Committee on Energy and Commerce, Subcommittee on Health and the Environment, December 15, 1981.

7. The president's budget totals assume Medicare savings from legislative and regulatory proposals, and offsetting premium contributions. Without these savings, Medicare's share would be somewhat lower in future years.

8. Karen Davis, "Recent Trends in Hospital Costs: Failure of the Voluntary Effort," testimony before the U.S. House of Representatives, Committee on Energy and Commerce, Subcommittee on Health and the Environment, December 15, 1981.

9. U.S. Department of Health and Human Services, National Center for Health Statistics, "Elderly People, the Population 65 Years and Over," in *Health, United States, 1976–1977* (Hyattsville, Md., 1977).

10. Congressional Budget Office, *Catastrophic Health Insurance* (Washington, D.C., January 1977).

11. James Luditz, Marian Gornick, and Ron Prihoda, *Use and Cost of Medicare Services in the Last Year of Life* (Baltimore: Health Care Financing Administration, September 21, 1981).

12. U.S. Department of Health and Human Services, National Center for Health Statistics, *Health, United States, 1981* (Hyattsville, Md., 1981).

13. Ida A. Merriam, testimony on Blue Cross and Other Private Health Insurance for the Elderly,

Hearings before the Subcommittee on Health of the Elderly of the Senate Special Committee on Aging, 88:2 (Washington, D.C.: U.S. Government Printing Office, 1964), pt. 1, 3–13.

14. Charles R. Fisher, "Difference by Age Groups in Health Care Spending," *Health Care Financing Review* (spring 1980).

15. U.S. Department of Health, Education, and Welfare, National Center for Health Statistics, *Personal Out-of-Pocket Health Expenses, United States, 1975,* series 10, no. 122.

16. Ronald Anderson et al., *Expenditures for Personal Health Services: National Trends and Variations, 1953–1970* (Washington, D.C.: Department of Health, Education and Welfare, 1973).

17. Regina Loewenstein, "The Effects of Medicare on the Health Care of the Aged," *Social Security Bulletin* (April 1971).

18. David F. Drake, "Does Money Spent on Health Care Really Improve U.S. Health Status?," *Hospitals* (October 16, 1978); and Avedis Donabedian, "Effects of Medicare and Medicaid on Access to and Quality of Health Care," *Public Health Reports* (July–August 1976).

19. U.S. Department of Health and Human Services, National Center for Health Statistics, *Current Estimates, 1980,* series 10, no. 139, and *Current Estimates, July 1963–June 1964,* series 10, no. 13.

20. Fisher, "Differences by Age Groups."

21. Bernard Friedman, "Mortality, Disability, and the Normative Economics of Medicare," in Richard N. Rossett, ed., *The Role of Health Insurance in the Health Services Sector* (Washington, D.C.: National Bureau of Economic Research, 1976).

22. *Health US, 1981.*

23. Ira Rosenwaike, Nurit Yaffe, and Phillip C. Sagi, "The Recent Decline in Mortality of the Extreme Aged: An Analysis of Statistical Data," *American Journal of Public Health* (October 1980).

24. Drake, "Money Spent on Health Care."

25. *Budget of the U.S. Government, FY 1983.*

26. Ibid.

27. Fisher, "Differences by Age Groups."

28. *Budget of the U.S. Government, FY 1983.*

29. Congressional Budget Office, "Reducing the Federal Deficit: Strategies and Options," February 5, 1982.

30. Ibid.

31. NCHS, *Current Estimates, 1980.*

32. U.S. Department of Commerce, Bureau of the Census, *Money Income and Poverty Status of Families and Persons in the United States, 1980,* series P-60, no. 127.

33. Joseph P. Newhouse et al., "Some Interim Results From a Controlled Trial of Cost Sharing in Health Insurance," *New England Journal of Medicine* (December 17, 1981).

34. Charles R. Link, Stephen H. Long, and Russell F. Settle, "Cost Sharing, Supplementary Insurance, and Health Services Utilization Among the Medicare Elderly," *Health Care Financing Review* (fall 1980).

35. U.S. Department of Commerce, Bureau of the Census, unpublished tables from the 1979 Current Population Survey.

36. For a description and analysis, see Glenn R. Markus, *Health Insurance: The Medicare Voucher Proposals* (Washington, D.C.: Congressional Research Service, December 10, 1981).

37. Disabled beneficiaries with renal dialysis would be retained in Medicare.

38. Markus, *Health Insurance.*

39. For a more complete discussion of the advantages of a voucher approach, see Paul Ginsburg, "Medicare Vouchers and the Procompetition Strategy," *Health Affairs* (winter 1981).

40. Ibid.

41. Fisher, "Differences by Age Groups."

42. Marjorie Muller et al., "Private Health Insurance Plans, 1977," *Health Care Financing Review.*

43. Burton E. Burton, senior vice-president, Aetna Life and Casualty, testimony before the U.S. House of Representatives, Ways and Means Subcommittee on Health, "Proposals to Stimulate Competition in the Financing and Delivery of Health Care," 97th Congress, 1st session, September 30–October 1, 1981; and Robert Helms, deputy assistant secretary for planning and evaluation/health, U.S. Department of Health and Human Services, personal communication.

44. U.S. House of Representatives, Select Committee on Aging, Hearings on Medi-Gap.

45. Senator Robert Dole, Remarks Before the American Hospital Association, February 1, 1982, Washington, D.C.

46. Congressional Budget Office, *Reducing the Federal Deficit: Strategies and Options* (Washington, D.C.: February 5, 1982).

47. John Holahan et al., "Paying for Physician Services under Medicare and Medicaid," *Milbank Memorial Fund Quarterly, Health and Society* (1979).

48. Statement of Senator Orrin Hatch, Final Consideration of S. 234, the Community Home Health Services Act, U.S. Senate Committee on Labor and Human Resources, December 15, 1981; and S. 234.

49. Alice Rivlin, letter to Senator Orrin Hatch, February 19, 1982.

50. White House, Office of the Press Secretary, *Fact Sheet, Federalism Initiative* (Washington, D.C.: January 27, 1982).

10. Response

Walter McNerney

Medicare has been a successful program, one of the best. It is the subject of intense scrutiny now because Washington is cost driven, and the cost of Medicare is large and growing rapidly. Cost sharing, however, has its limits, no matter how we feel about it. It hits a selected population hard, and most of these people are deeply interested in security, so that the ability of society to transfer costs to the individual has practical limits.

I agree that there are a lot of problems with vouchers, and I believe that utilization review, about to be discontinued under PSRO, needs a replacement. Further, I agree that we have to move to incentive reimbursement and that we need to broaden benefits.

What should we do next? There is a lack of consensus in both the private and public sectors. In early 1981, everybody thought that through consumer choice, option, and some competition we could come up with a good system that would favorably affect not only the private sector, but the public sector as well. It was clear that the system was not working very well; there was reduced entry, efficient and inefficient providers got paid equally, there was restricted choice, etc. The more this debate unfolded, the more it became clear that there were a lot of problems involved in the practical implementation of these ideas. As Dr. Ginzberg said earlier, now is not the time to act impulsively. Now is the time to build some consensus and to act a little more reflectively.

In the short run I would suggest that the government take a very careful look at cost shifting. It is very likely that if it continues unabated it could seriously fragment the system and antagonize people to the point that some bad decisions might be made. The government should also get out of the niggling business, for example, the two percent arbitrary unsupported reduction in hospital costs.

Now is not the time to repeal the Planning Act. We are going to need a forum for consensus building and for molding public and professional opinion. The coalitions are too untried, untested and too frail to take on planning. We must get a substitute for PSRO because some very quick decisions, neglecting quality, can be made and checks are needed. I, personally, would lay out review standards that would have to be met by providers and would be less involved in precisely how they were met.

This is a timely moment to get into incentive reimbursement, for there is a quiet revolution underway in the delivery of care. The horizontal and vertical integration now underway in the health field is nothing short of dramatic; there is ferment; there is a demonstrated willingness to experiment. Packaging of these new ventures, including but not confined to HMOs, with different pricing is appropriate. We must stop thinking of HMOs as the only imaginative alternatives. There are many other ways that care can be packaged.

In the short run we must also look at disability. I think the doubtful claims here are much more extensive than people recognize. Further, if we do not broaden benefits, we are going to put excessive pressure on the hospital at great expense. I would suggest trading hospital days for home care or other alternatives to the hospital.

It would be good to develop a more sophisticated relationship with intermediaries, meaning greater reference to standards and objectives and less meddling in the administrative processes. Under the CHAMPUS program, there was a period of experimentation with bidding by intermediaries to save money and enlarge competition. Blue Cross and Blue Shield entered that period with 30 percent of the business and emerged with 80 percent.

Importantly, the problems of the aging cannot be divorced from their social and political context; we have to be concerned with total lifestyle and with an overall public policy. Our current perspective is too narrow.

11. Response

Lynn Etheredge

Dr. Davis' paper gives us both the background of the Medicare program and an overview of different savings opportunities. When talking about savings, we need to keep in mind the enormous size of the Medicare program. During the 1980s the federal government will spend $750 billion on Medicare. I think major dollar savings can be made in the program without having to cut back on basic benefits to those in need. Even one percent of that $750 billion is a very substantial amount of money.

Dr. Davis pointed out that a $1 billion annual reduction has already resulted from the 1981 Economic Reconciliation Act. The administration's 1982 proposals are for $3 billion of savings in the first year. Taken together, those proposals alone would probably save $60 billion in the rest of this decade.

If you look over Dr. Davis' list of the administration's proposals, I suggest you will discover that they fit within the charge that Dr. Rogers put to everyone —to try to find ways to economize in government spending that do not harm basic benefits or deny needed services. For example, indexing the Part B deductible to the consumer price index will save $65 million next year, but that index is the same as for Social Security benefits, so the deductible will grow with the ability to pay the deductible. That will save $2 billion over the rest of the decade.

A 5 percent coinsurance for home health services is another such change. Home health spending is now over $1 billion and growing over 30 percent a year, with no cost sharing at all. Costs next year will be $48 a visit compared with $65 for an average day in a nursing home. A 5 percent copayment, $2.40, is unlikely to deny needed benefits. You may not like this particular list of niggardly proposals, but such nickels and dimes in a $750 billion program add up to very real savings and are essential if we are going to avoid major cuts in basic benefits.

For the future, the administration is developing proposals to strengthen health sector competition. The president has decided that he is serious about not wanting to increase taxes, even through the back door, by limiting employer health insurance contributions. He has also decided that he does not like new regulation of employers. As a result, the administration may wind up proposing a voluntary program of expanded employee plan offerings.

The major Medicare procompetition proposal being considered is a voucher system which, as Dr. Ellwood has described, may contain major savings opportunities. Dr. Davis has summarized a number of the technical problems that need to be resolved. In principle, I think that the problems of designing a voucher system are solvable. The skewed distribution of expenditures for the Medicare population is the same as for the under sixty-five population. Private insurance has solved those problems for decades.

Dr. Davis suggests some ways in which further reductions can be made in the Medicare program while preserving its basic benefits and helping to cope with massive budget deficits. I think the figures she presented demonstrate that the most important element of a Medicare budget strategy has to be to reduce cigarette consumption and alcohol abuse.

With 9 percent of the aged using 70 percent of the health care, at an average cost of $7,000; with 3.5 percent of the population under sixty-five consuming 50 percent of the health care every year; with 75 percent of the aged dying from heart disease, cancer, and cerebrovascular disease, I see nothing that will have a bigger payoff in terms of the Medicare budget—and health status—than being able to make substantial reductions in alcohol consumption and cigarette use. The recent surgeon general's report calls for a much stronger cigarette labeling requirement and the authority of the secretary to specify what label goes on what cigarette. Serious consideration should also be given to tripling alcohol and tobacco taxes, which would raise $15 billion a year, and simply index those taxes to increasing inflation since they were last raised in the 1950s.

A second area in which major savings can be made is physician reimbursement. I agree with Dr. Davis that Medicare's payment system is long overdue for overhaul, but I do not think we ought to replace usual and customary fees with negotiated fee schedules for two reasons. First, I don't think such fee schedules would work very well. No physician organization represents most physicians, and those that do represent physicians do not have the authority to negotiate binding fee schedules. More importantly, such an arrangement would encourage physicians to band together to fix prices, which would probably drive prices up in the long run. Second, I think the physician market is now made to order for vigorous price cutting and cost control through competition, particularly as we get further into the 1980s and there is an oversupply of physicians, especially in the overpriced specialties. Physician fees may now be a house of cards supported only by an outdated third-party reimbursement method.

We should be able to find ways to exploit the physician supply situation and save billions of dollars, perhaps paying physicians $100 more if they will do surgery on an outpatient basis, cutting the 20 percent Medicare coinsurance for physicians with lower fees or requesting that physicians submit competitive bids for setting Medicare reimbursement rates. This is a situation in which we can take advantge of the market situation without denying benefits.

With respect to hospital care, the administration is working on prospective budgeting proposals. Competition theorists have argued that some forms of prospective budgeting are undesirable since they restrict freedom of entry and the ability of lower cost providers to compete. To my mind, prospective budgeting and competition can be reconciled, for example, through Section 223 limits, which set a maximum reimbursement for hospitals but allow lower cost institutions to fully and vigorously compete and to grow.

There are also major savings opportunities in utilization review, if we can find ways to capitalize on them. One of the few statistics not mentioned in Dr. Davis' presentation is that Medicare lengths of stay consistently run 50 percent higher in the Northeast than on the West Coast, even after adjusting for age and sex of patient, diagnosis, and procedure. We simply cannot afford to continue to pay for patterns that do not have any justification, and neither can private employers. The medical community needs to find ways for the government to assure appropriate care without wasting resources. I do not think it is yet time to propose again a regional medical program for heart, cancer, and stroke patients, but those are areas I would target for additional studies, to see if we can find ways to both improve health and hold down expenses.

12. Response

Paul Rogers

Mr. Etheredge's proposal to put more taxes on alcohol and tobacco to help rationalize any cuts and perhaps prevent further cuts in health care expenditures will be seriously considered by Congress.

The 1981 cuts in Medicare probably got through Congress more easily because they were handled by a procedure that Congress is unfamiliar with, the Budget Reconciliation Act. I doubt if those cuts would have gotten through if they had gone through the usual legislative process. Congress will probably be unable to use that same mechanism as effectively another time because some of the legislative committees are going to assert themselves a little more than they did before. Although there may be some cuts, I am not sure they will be of the same magnitude as last year's.

Prospective budgeting will probably be tried, but that is just a new name for cost controls.

I do think that Congress is going to be interested in new forms of delivery. Congress has already supported HMOs, and I think encouragement will be given to day surgery centers and home health care. There will probably be reimbursement for home health care and support for hospices to decrease the high cost of dying. Home health care may be more expensive at first, until we learn how to handle it, just like any new technology.

One area that we have not talked about that needs consideration is research. As the federal government reduces support for research, I think the private sector, including organizations like the American Hospital Association, the AMA, the HCA, and so forth, ought to be giving some thought to how we can encourage research in areas where advances could dramatically reduce cost and relieve some of the suffering of the elderly.

Discussion

Dr. Ginzberg: We appear to agree that the health care services provided to the poor and elderly under Medicaid and Medicare are now vulnerable. Some states are now severely restricting access to nursing homes and the days of care that they will provide. The large teaching hospitals that care for large numbers of the inner city poor are concerned about how they are going to continue treating those patients. Once the federal government says to the states, "You go and buy your Medicaid services at whatever rate you like competitively!" we are going to be in a very difficult situation because those large teaching hospitals cannot compete.

I have read that many municipal and county hospitals are being sold to for-profit chains. These hospitals are easy for governments in some parts of the country to sell, and they seem to be attractive to the for-profit chains. As I understand it, these sales mean that governments are trying in different ways to cut their commitments to the poor, to get themselves in the position of not having to respond.

If the business coalitions ever get serious, one item high on their agenda ought to be joint approaches to sharing the unpaid bills that result from the treatment of the poor who are uninsured or only partly insured.

We have kept the system going these last years with cross subsidization. But, if that is reaching its limits and if nonprofit urban hospitals serving large numbers of the poor are going to have to compete on price with suburban, frequently proprietary hospitals treating very few of the poor, how will we cope with this kind of market segmentation without full reimbursement of services to the poor?

Mr. MacNaughton: It is true that many community hospitals are now approaching the for-profit hospital groups. In fact, we have more proposals than we want to entertain. Many come from places where we could never invest because there is no way that their hospitals could break even. Newark, New Jersey, is a perfect example. Their community hospitals cannot possibly make it financially, unless their patients are fully subsidized.

But there are a lot of other community hospitals that are finding it very difficult to break even, despite a large amount of business that is subsidized by the community. We are interested in these hospitals because we see ways of making them turn a profit. They do not make a profit before we come in, for many reasons. One is inefficiency. Often, for example, we find they do not even pick up the reimbursements to which they are entitled. One lost a million dollars last year, and neglected to claim two million dollars worth of reimbursements.

Another reason is politics, especially in the municipal and county hospitals Dr. Ginzberg mentioned. A lot of the people who work in public hospitals are there not for hospital reasons but for political reasons, and city councillors and county supervisors are frequently anxious to get rid of that system. Often when we bid for these hospitals we are the lowest bidder, but we still get the business because we approach them on this basis: "You have a large indigent population. The more you charge us, the more we have to pay for the hospital, the higher our rates have to be in order to finance this purchase. You're not selling the hospital to hurt the residents of your community; you're selling it to help them. Why don't you take the lowest bidder? Furthermore, what are you going to do with the several millions of dollars we'll pay you for your hospital? Why don't you put that in a fund for indigents because that would be a good and appropriate way to use the money?"

Often they accept our reasoning. But we almost always have to promise that anybody who comes to that hospital will be cared for after we have acquired it.

Mr. Califano: I think that dotting the i's and crossing the t's on the reimbursement regulations is critical. The reality is that people want to get every possible dollar of reimbursement. Those who write the regulations are having an enormous impact on the health care system. The questions they answer never reach an assistant secretary or deputy secretary.

People know how Part A and Part B of Medicare work and how Medicaid works, and how to handle patients. Doctors, particularly groups like radiologists and cardiologists, are increasingly working out deals with hospitals in the context of Part A and Part B and Medicaid. HMOs are now functioning on a fee-for-service basis for Medicaid and Medicare patients, getting what they can out of state reimbursement or the private insurance companies. Somehow we must come to understand that all of this is related and put it together. That is part of the reason why Medicare and Medicaid will ultimately have to be combined in one system.

Dr. Sammons: It disturbs us a great deal that freedom of choice is beginning to disappear from Medicaid. There is something inherently dishonest about promising the American public freedom of choice in the 1960s and then taking it away in the 1980s. If you look at the reimbursement mechanisms, you see that neither of the federal programs is paying its share and that a significant number of doctors and a significant number of hospitals simply don't want to treat Medicaid and Medicare beneficiaries. We have doctors in this country who say, "I'll either treat them for free or not at all because it's too much trouble and it costs too much and it's too cumbersome to try and get reimbursed!"

The federal government continues to cut back the percentage of reimbursement for usual, customary, and reasonable fees in the Medicare program. One or two years from now I suspect we will be talking about how you get providers to treat the poor and elderly.

We have an ever-increasing number of elderly, and the vast majority of them are not poor. They have worked for forty-five years in the most productive and the most affluent period of American history. The presumption that they are poor simply because they have reached the chronological age of sixty-five is nonsense, but we have built a system on that theory. We must put some reason back into this.

There seems to be a rationale among those who administer Medicare and Medicaid that says you don't pay the usual, customary, and reasonable fees, but at the same time you expect hospitals and physicians to accept patients for whatever Medicare and Medicaid will pay. You don't have to be a mathematical genius to figure out that a doctor is not going to do that, nor can you expect hospitals to continue the cost shift.

The underlying thesis that there is something terribly wrong with the system is foolishness. There's nothing really wrong with the system that time and the system itself can't straighten out. The time has come for some reason to be applied to the problem, instead of a lot of rhetoric. When I look at the available dollars and at the loss of freedom of choice, I worry about how long it will be before Medicare recipients are told that freedom of choice is no longer available to them, either.

Dr. Nesbitt: During Mr. Califano's tenure with HEW he appointed a committee to study the manpower issues in this country. I served with that group for its full four-and-a-half years. I think that there was one overriding element of the report of that committee that has a heavy impact on what we are talking about. Certainly, the report heightened society's understanding of the expansion of the physician supply. I think it is terribly important that we understand that for the decade of the eighties there is not a single thing that we are going to do that will alter the annual addition to the manpower pool of about 17,000 new physicians. The most important aspect of that whole report, however, is what happens in the decade of the nineties. Between 1990 and 2000, we will expand the physician supply far beyond our greatest expectations. The reason that is important is its impact on our academic health centers. That is where the expense of training these individuals rests and these academic health centers are going to be facing tremendous financial burdens. As they look at cost issues and the steps they must take to control those costs, it becomes fairly clear that a number of training programs will be subject to reduction.

We are also facing some difficulty in meeting the needs of the current crop of physicians for training programs as they graduate. Today there are no extra slots, partly because of U.S. citizens training in the foreign schools.

I take a different view from Dr. Sammons about physicians' willingness to participate in Medicare and Medicaid in the years ahead. I think we will find that in some areas they are going to be willing to take whatever patients they can find in order to practice medicine. The positions of many physicians will be modified as they look at the amount and sources of their income, and at the shrinking percentage that comes from other sources.

Dr. Nelson: I think that the distribution of access may change, but that the poor will get the care they need.

Mr. MacNaughton: I think it depends on where you are. The access for the big city poor will be less. For the rural poor, access will hold steady or improve.

Mr. McNerney: As I said yesterday, society is going to be sorely tempted to take it out on those who can defend themselves the least. But I don't think the reductions are going to be significant. I think the change will be marginal.

Dr. Ginzberg: Since the urban poor get so much of their service from the emergency rooms and clinics of the hospitals, you have to allow time for the hospitals to get into major trouble. Only then will you see the impact of the reductions. It will take a few more years for us to discover what the word "significant" really means.

Dr. Cooper: I don't agree with Dr. Nesbitt about the physician supply. The number is still going up, but we are going to be able to train and employ them. They may not be in the hospital they want to be in, but we are still going to be able to take care of three or more years of residency training.

The problem in this country is that the number of public general hospital beds has been decreasing substantially in relationship to the population. Philadelphia doesn't even have one. Cook County Hospital used to have 3,500 beds; it now has 750 beds. If we have a lot of these hospitals taken over by the proprietary chains, there will be a problem.

The academic medical centers, where the poor and elderly now go, are simply not going to be able to take care of them. Already some of these hospitals, in order to survive, are beginning to say, "We can't take care of them!" It's a rapidly changing situation because the places that have always cared for these people are simply not going to be able to do it anymore.

In Washington, D.C., physicians are becoming very cautious about changing fees, and about the patients that they will and will not see, because Washington has the highest proportion of physicians to population in the United States. A new physician simply can't operate in that city anymore, and existing physicians are having trouble maintaining their incomes.

Dr. Nelson: All of us will eventually go through an interval between the time we become eligible for Medicare and the time we die, during which time we will consume services. Some of those services are expensive, and some of them are not. One of the things we really have not looked at very much is the impact of the disease mix that we experience during that time interval.

For instance, it is relatively inexpensive for us to die of coronary artery disease, because 40 percent of us die before we make it to the hospital. As a matter of fact, if we are successful in eliminating coronary artery disease, expenditures for Medicare will go up because people will live longer and die of some infinitely messier, more expensive disease, like cancer. I think the disease mix and its impact on total health expenditures is something we are going to have to look at.

Prof. Mechanic: I think Dr. Sammons' statement is as strong a statement for national health insurance as any I have ever heard.

We have a public system, but we try to disguise it as a private system. The incompatibility between the public system and the masquerade creates lots of problems, so we apply regulations and they are very unproductive. Given the number of old people and the number of doctors, and the resistance to increased taxes for Social Security, the government is going to have difficulty in carrying its share.

We see cost shifting in lots of sectors; in the universities, for example, where it costs far more to train a student in physics than in political science, though they pay the same tuition. We don't complain very much about cost shifting in that setting.

Looking at the campaign that has been mounted against cost shifting in reponse to the cutbacks in Medicare, I think the message is very clear that the private sector is not willing to live under any rules other than the traditional rules of reimbursement, unless it is forced to do so.

What is the value of putting the scalpel to Medicare compared with asking whether we really need $200 billion of new capital investment as the private sector claims, when that is largely an investment for the affluent and not for the poor. It seems to me that we are at an impasse. We are in a situation of rationing. If we are going to ration, perhaps we ought to think about it carefully and examine its effects. As I see the system evolving now, the people who will bear the brunt of rationing will be the poor and the old people with lower incomes. There are smaller groups that are going to suffer worse, however; one such group is the chronic mentally ill. They are at the bottom of this totem pole, and they are going to get pushed out of the system entirely.

Prof. Joseph Lipscomb, Jr.: I just want to comment very briefly on some areas that take us beyond Medicare and Medicaid but relate to alternative approaches to care for the elderly. I am talking in particular about the sort of policies, perhaps tax policies, that would induce the elderly to make decisions earlier in their life cycle that would make it much easier for them to provide for their own health, safety, and social welfare in their older years. I am talking about policies that would lead to a rationalization of pension plans with Social Security, private health insurance, and public health insurance.

By examining the tax code, we could determine how changes might be made to affect who saves and how much is saved, how much health insurance is bought, and affecting those who hire and fire people and when that choice occurs. I am talking about tax changes that might induce others to take care of the elderly in ways that are currently not being done. Subtle tax changes might lead to long-run changes in the savings behavior of individuals, the hiring behavior of firms, and the amount of welfare that is provided by the private sector to the elderly.

Dr. DuVal: I would like to make three observations. First, as long as the medical profession works in a medium that is so complex that it is not understood by the patient, and as long as the largest purchaser of medical services is the public dollar, ultimately it is in the best interest of the medical profession to assure the decision makers who control the public dollar that what they are doing is necessary and that the service is rendered at the right level. The greatest mistake that we have made in medicine is to abandon fee-for-service.

Second, I do not think that prospective reimbursement should be misrepresented. It is being sold as a cost control device, put in place for the purpose of achieving efficiency. It is in fact a rationing device, and it should not be disguised as something else. It is a device for transferring from the public to a specific profession responsibility for decisions about which services will be rendered and which will not.

Third, is it not likely that the escalation of costs and insurance payouts is reaching the point where there will be more and more self-insurance and where some insurance companies will be put into a position where they cannot sell insurance anymore?

Prof. Davis: Mr. Etheredge defended the administration's FY 1983 Medicare reduction proposals by pointing out that, while they may look like nickel-and-dime economies, they generate $60 billion in savings over a decade and that they represent only small cuts relative to the total outlays for Medicare. According to my estimates, the Medicare savings proposals included in last year's Reconciliation Act, this year's budget, and the promised future Medicare legislation, would represent 20 percent of Medicare payments after five years. That is a substantial cut even relative to the size of the Medicare program. Those kinds of cuts are going to be an enormous economic burden, particularly on the lower income elderly who do not have supplemental private health insurance. Are there better alternatives to these cuts? I think the Ways and Means Committee's rejection of those proposals indicates that Congress certainly thinks there are.

There is no excuse for not moving to more fundamental reimbursement reform. We are in a situation of extraordinarily rapid increases in health care costs. Since Congress voted not to cap hospital costs, they have accelerated markedly; the rate of increase is currently running at a 19 to 20 percent annual rate. That wreaks havoc on Medicare, since 70 percent of its expenditures is for hospital services.

There are two possible approaches to this problem. One is to do something about health care costs directly through a cost containment approach. The other is simply for each payer to try to reduce the share of the total he pays, and I think that is what we are seeing in these policies.

We are on a collision course, with federal, state, and local governments trying to cut health expenditures in the face of very rapid inflation in the health sector. Those who are going to be hurt in the collision are the poor and the elderly, who are going to have more of the cost shifting back onto them directly.

I think it is important to have a unified policy. Federalizing Medicare and merging it with Medicaid, having a single reimbursement policy across those two programs, would be helpful, but it has to include the private insurers as well. Dr. Sammons' point about the federal government not paying its share is true. It is going to be even more true in the future if we do not get a unified reimbursement policy.

Dr. DuVal's point that we shouldn't misrepresent prospective reimbursement is also true. Prospective reimbursement differs from cost containment in that we are not just talking about limits on rates of increase over time. We are talking about a rational way of paying providers, so that all providers providing the same service would be paid the same rate. We are a long way from that now. For example, if you take hospitals of a given size, adjust for the fact that they are in different wage areas, and adjust for the fact that they have different mixes of patients, you will still find that their costs per admission range from $1,000 to $3,000. For Medicare or private insurers to pay rates that differ by as much as $2,000, simply because those are the actual costs, is inequitable, inefficient, and the wrong way to go.

Prospective reimbursement addresses that issue, but it is not just a matter of trying to get a more equitable or efficient reimbursement system. It is also giving payers a say in what the rate increases will be over time. That involves putting responsibility on health providers to live within total limits, but I think that is part of the negotiation process. I don't think it has to mean rationing in the sense of cutting out essential services.

Dr. Sammons' position on freedom of choice is one that I share. Both of us wrote letters to every member of the Senate urging the defeat of limitation of freedom of choice under Medicaid. I frequently argue in cases like this that you should not be willing to support policies for the poor that you would be unwilling to advocate for the elderly. It troubles me that we would tell the poor that a state has the right to decide which physicians they may go to, which hospitals they may or may not be admitted to, both because it affects access to care and because it interferes with the right of patients to select their own provider. If Medicare keeps cutting reimbursement for providers, whether physicians or hospitals, providers are going to be unwilling to take those patients and, therefore, even the elderly will be faced with a situation of not being able to choose freely.

My next point is about Medicare vouchers. Mr. Etheredge said that there is an uneven distribution of expenditures for medical care among the nonelderly and that private insurance companies have coped with that for decades; therefore, there is no reason for Medicare vouchers not to work if there is a similar skew of those expenditures among the elderly. The way the private insurance sector has coped with this is called experience rating, which is very different from a fixed voucher amount. In fact, Medicare is experienced rated. It basically pays the expenditures and hires insurers to pay the claims due to administrative prices on top of that. There is a fundamental flaw in the Medicare voucher idea, however, and that is adverse risk selection. So far, I see no way around that problem, given the skewing of expenditures. I think we should be wary about moving in that direction.

There have been a number of good comments about the physician supply. Mr. Etheredge said he thought that the big increase in physicians over the decade was going to cause price competition and lower fees. Therefore, we should not change our reimbursement policy in the area of physician's services because it might interfere with the desire on the part of the physicians to undercut each other and get more business by lowering their fees. I have looked at areas that are clearly saturated with physicians, areas with an average supply, and areas with a shortage of physicians. I found that physicians' fees are higher in areas with more physicians. Incomes are lower, though. While physicians charge higher fees in those areas, they are not able to generate sufficient volume to keep their incomes up. In areas with more physicians, health care costs and utilization are much higher, hospital admission rates are much higher, lengths of stay are longer, and hospital costs per day are a lot higher. Medicare physician expenditures for enrollees are a lot higher. So this enormous explosion of physician supply will cause much greater expenditures for both hospitals and physician services. I project that the increase in physician supply over the 1980s will increase health expenditures by $50 billion by 1990.

I agree with Dr. Nesbitt that there is not much that we can do about the supply of physicians now in medical school. We do need to begin to think about policies to affect the supply between 1990 and 2000 and to determine how to get the most out of this increased supply. How can we get more physicians in rural or inner city areas? How can we get more of them serving the poor? While I think there is going to be competition for patients, I doubt that the competition will lead to services for those who cannot pay unless we have some positive policies. This increase in physicians provides an enormous opportunity if we are willing to try to redirect that supply or take advantage of it. It might cost more but we will get more benefit out of it if we plan.

We should focus some attention and research on the 9 percent of the Medicare population that accounts for 70 percent of the expenditures. The basic data source is the Medicare claims file that gives information on age of patients, types of services, procedures, etc., but so far those data have not been analyzed. There is some suggestion that Medicare use can be predicted by utilization in the previous year. There is a recurring pattern of very strong utilizers, chronically ill individuals who must use the health care system year after year. I think we need to find out a lot more about that population, what kinds of medical problems they have, how they are occurring, what kinds of services they receive, and what kind of procedures they undergo. The results might indicate avenues for private medical research that would have high payoff as well.

My final comments have to do with the poor elderly and access to care. In 1980 the median income of the elderly was $4,225. That is above the federally defined poverty level, but it is not a high income. The bulk of the elderly have reasonably low income, and their economic situation is aggravated by two factors: first, high inflation, which has eroded the savings of the elderly and, second, increases in life expectancy, which means that whatever accumulation of wealth they have must sustain them over a longer lifetime.

The cutbacks in Medicaid have resulted in large numbers of individuals being dropped from the Medicaid rolls. In the last couple of years, we have lost several million people from Medicaid simply because the states have not been increasing eligibility levels.

I think we are going to see more closings of public clinics and municipal hospitals. Teaching hospitals that have never denied admission to anyone who couldn't pay must now rethink their admission policies. Hearings last year by the Oversight Committee of the House Energy and Commerce Committee documented case after case of individuals turned away from hospitals simply because the patients couldn't come up with $500 preadmission deposits. These kinds of things are going to accelerate.

We know now that two-thirds of the poor are not on Medicaid. That is a fraction that will grow because of the cutbacks. The uninsured use physician services half as much as the insured. The insured have two-and-a-half times as much possible care as the uninsured. Coverage and ability to pay make an enormous difference here. The health problems of the uninsured are greater than those of the insured so that, after adjusting for health needs, one finds even greater disparities.

There is a new survey by the Office of Civil Rights and the Department of Health and Human Services on race and source of payment of hospital patients. It shows which hospitals take the uninsured poor, which ones take the Medicaid patients, and which ones take the Medicare patients. Among the 160 largest public hospitals, the uninsured represent 37 percent of the total patient population, privately insured patients represent about 20 percent, and the rest are on public programs, Medicare and Medicaid. Among for-profit hospitals 4 percent of the patients are uninsured poor, over half are privately insured, and the rest are on Medicare and Medicaid. Hospitals that take care of the uninsured poor are experiencing serious financial strain. With many of them being public institutions, and with the budgetary cutbacks we all expect, I think access to care will become increasingly difficult.

13. Financial Support of Health Care of the Elderly and the Indigent: Institutions Likely to Be at Risk and Solutions

Perhaps the most important question for domestic public policy of this decade is how to provide high quality health care to all our citizens at a cost we can afford. Left unchecked, rising health care costs could consume virtually all our resources. Improbable as that event may be, efforts to keep these expenditures in some acceptable relationship to other parts of our economy have met with only limited success. It is quite clear that we are living in a cost-driven society. Even economists will say that they do not know if health care costs should absorb 9, 10, or 15 percent of the Gross National Product. One example of the seriousness of the situation we now face is that Prudential Life Insurance Company recently discontinued selling health insurance to individuals.

The major reasons for increasing health care costs are familiar to us all: labor intensive hospitals, innovative and expensive technology, a permissive reimbursement system, lack of competition, and an increasingly older population. Of these, the elderly, coupled with the indigent population, will assume an increasingly important role through time. First, they are major consumers of federal dollars. Over $66 billion was spent for Medicare and Medicaid in 1981, representing approximately 25 percent of all dollars spent for health care in the United States. Second, while states have variable commitments to Medicaid, higher taxes are bringing heavy political pressures on elected officials to keep Medicaid expenditures level, or even reduce them. Third, as our population ages, we should expect greater expenditures to apply our vast array of technology to the treatment of the multi-system diseases that characteristically affect the elderly, the indigent, and the handicapped.

As resources to support health care shrink relative to demand, our society will face some difficult choices. These issues will include questions about who shall live and who shall die, questions dealing with access and ability to pay, the kind of system we want (pluralistic vs. government controlled), how we pay for it all, and how we preserve those institutions at risk in an era of increasingly limited resources.

Institutions at Risk

The tertiary care hospital. Of the institutions at greatest risk, the tertiary care hospital is the most vulnerable because of its high cost. Most commonly located in an urban setting with a large elderly and indigent population, it is committed, indeed expected, to devote its high cost technology to serve the neediest population (e.g., those suffering trauma, burns, heart disease, cancer, stroke). In some instances, such technologic capacity must be provided on a standby basis (e.g., burns or neonatology), thus incurring expense without offsetting revenue. Such hospitals usually operate active emergency and outpatient services that are vital to the community needs but far from fiscally self-sustaining. Furthermore, not only because of their more limited technologic capacity, but also to avoid treating high cost illnesses, suburban or rural hospitals may refer patients to the tertiary hospital for treatment of the final (and often most costly) stages of their illness. Such referrals are made from doctor to doctor. Responsibility for accepting patients resides in the individual physician, who is unaffected by the fiscal problems of the hospital since he assumes no risk by accepting the patient for treatment. Occasionally, no consultation takes place at all; the patient is simply delivered by ambulance to the tertiary care hospital, because its policy to accept all patients needing therapy is well known.

A similar tactic may be employed by nursing homes that want to dispose of a patient. The patient is taken to the hospital emergency room, the nursing home bed is filled by another patient, and the hospital must admit a patient who inevitably becomes a placement problem. In such circumstances, the hospital is acting as a nursing home, depriving potential patients of much needed treatment, and often receiving inadequate reimbursement for the inappropriately occupied bed.

Finally, tertiary care hospitals are usually committed to residency training programs to varying degrees. Such programs have both educational and service components. While these components contribute to the high cost of hospitalization, such costs might be even greater were paramedical or other special personnel employed to carry out the service function that residents perform while working longer hours and at lower pay. Ironically, the success of the residency programs of many institutions has led their graduates to locate in nearby institutions and compete for patients with the organizations that trained them (although such competition has not produced lower costs).

Compounding the difficulties of the tertiary care hospitals are the proprietary chains and HMO-owned hospitals, which employ modern management techniques and skim the lower risk, less sick patients from the patient population. They are able to operate at lower cost, and they are gaining an increasing market share.

Thus, the tertiary care hospital is most vulnerable during these times because it is losing its ability to maintain a balance between the technological characteristics of an intensive care unit and those required to treat the less seriously ill patients. The tertiary care hospital is at risk of becoming only an intensive care unit with a major component of its patients being elderly, indigent or both. In such circumstances, the cost of care will escalate far above its present level and in all likelihood prove unacceptable to the third-party payers. A logical step would then be to cap the costs, thus reducing the capability of the hospital to provide sophisticated tertiary care and stifling innovation and medical education.

While these observations apply to both private- and city-operated tertiary care hospitals, history is proving that the American city, particularly in the Northeast, does not wish to maintain a high cost, high technology facility. Rather, to the extent that the city stays in the hospital business, it will provide a "safety net" for its citizens. High technology medicine will be provided by the private sector on a self-referral basis or through the occasional contractual relationship where funding is available.

Neighborhood or rural health centers. Most of these centers started in the early 1970s with encouragement from the federal government to provide health services to the underserved and the indigent. Some were free standing while others were affiliated with or direct operating extensions of hospital centers. Over time, the majority of such centers have shut their doors, due to poor management, withdrawal of funding, loss of patients, or a combination of these factors. Most of the remaining centers represent that group closely tied to major hospital centers. They have survived because of the financial underpinning the parent hospital has provided. The hospital, commonly teaching and tertiary in character, benefits from patient referral, residency training, and maintaining good relations with its neighborhood. However, few such health centers can pay their own way and must depend on special government programs and the hospital for support. Many such clinics treat both the indigent and the elderly, and a diminution in support from direct patient revenue, from the reduction of targeted federal programs or from the parent hospital, will place them in jeopardy.

Medical schools. Many medical schools do not own or operate their teaching hospitals, but others have direct operating authority, with all the attendant benefits and problems. Unfortunately, in recent years the operating budgets of the hospital and medical school have far exceeded those of the parent university. Further, the atmosphere and operating style of an academic institution is quite different from that of a hospital. While the academic intellectual and the practitioner have much in common, opportunities to emphasize their differences arise all the time. For example, university and hospital salary scales for professional and nonprofessional personnel are difficult, if not impossible, to reconcile. In the relationship between university and hospital there is often an uneasy truce at many levels with the potential for significant disagreement, particularly at the faculty level. The medical school often sees a portion of its financial salvation deriving from the practices of hospital-based physicians, a view accepted by deans and preclinical faculty, but not so enthusiastically by the fund-generating clinical faculty.

The institutional risk accrues to medical schools and their universities both educationally and financially if the scenario described above for the tertiary care hospital occurs. In such a circumstance, the university would be at considerable financial risk, the medical school would lose the type of hospital necessary to train its students and residents, and the faculty as a whole could be fragmented and left to argue why the situation was ever allowed to occur in the first place.

Possible Solutions

Any approach to dealing with such a complex set of issues is multifaceted and must be adaptable to the special needs of a given situation. For example, Duke University Hospital and the hospitals affiliated with Harvard have much in common educationally, but they have substantial differences in their relations with their universities, their fiscal operations, and the populations they serve. Nonetheless, the following suggestions are generic and systemic approaches to dealing with the problems posed not only by our commitment to care for the elderly and the indigent, but also by our concern to provide a suitable structure in which to care for all.

First, the business of the hospital must be defined. What does it want to be? Does it want to emphasize a balance of services across the board, or does it want to exclude specialties such as obstetrics, pediatrics, and eye, ear, nose and throat? Does it want to emphasize burn care, cardiovascular surgery, etc? Does it have a way of measuring the success of its business (surgery, medicine, psychiatry, etc), and do the doctors feel they have a personal stake in the success of that business? Human nature responds to incentives, both negative and positive, and the motivation of the physician is critical to the success of whatever business the hospital chooses to be in.

Second, once the business is defined and the caretakers are committed to it both personally and institutionally, the hospital can manage and market its products with the expectation that it can deliver a quality product in a timely manner to individuals or groups (corporations, unions, schools, etc.). Any arrangement should be entered into with a commitment to maintain a blend of patients with high and low cost illnesses. The proper blend allows the hospital to subsidize treatment of the more costly illnesses through the appropriate charge structure and to maintain the balance necessary to the mental health of the staff of a tertiary hospital (witness the difficulty in staffing intensive care units). In the teaching hospital, this patient mix provides the type of experience essential to the training of modern physicians.

Third, intrinsic to this process is the need for monitoring intake of patients, particularly those referred from outlying hospitals, to ensure their admission is appropriate. For patients hopelessly ill, admission obviously is not indicated, but conveying the negative answer in a manner that does not cut off further referrals requires consummate diplomatic skill. Yet refusing the patient is in the best interest of the patient, the tertiary hospital, and the fiscal intermediary.

Similar considerations apply to withholding heroic measures from patients entering the hospital directly with hopeless medical situations, for example, the elderly patient with a leaking aortic aneurysm, diabetes, and renal failure. The same factors apply to the hospitalized patient who has become hopelessly ill. In this situation, caretakers often disagree about what to do. Asking the advice of a group of medical experts and lay people may make the doctor and family's decision about the appropriateness of further therapy much easier.

In both circumstances the guiding principle is the practice of high quality medicine which requires the application of therapy where indicated and withholding or withdrawal when further treatment would only add to pain and suffering—and unnecessary utilization of resources which could be more effectively applied to other patients.

Fourth, medicine by nature is inefficient; paradoxically, it has been made more so by the technological explosion of the past twenty years. Thus it has been said that we must learn to govern our technology rather than have it govern us. This is particularly true in the tertiary hospital, where all kinds of technology are available. Use of technology consistent with good medical practice is an important and practical means of conserving resources. Every hospital could be more efficient in minimizing length of stay and performing only those tests and procedures absolutely necessary for diagnosis and therapy. Peer review is clearly the only effective and sensible way of bringing this about.

Fifth, discharge planning should begin at the time of hospital admission, particularly for elderly patients, who often have no relatives in the area and no permanent home. Traditional placement in a nursing home may not be possible or desirable, and alternatives such as elder care, foster care, or entry into a life care center should be explored. Early discharge planning has the obvious advantage of keeping length of stay to a minimum, thus utilizing resources of the hospital and fiscal intermediary most effectively.

In considering opportunities to conserve or generate resources outside the mainstream of patient care, several avenues are worth pursuing. First is the continuing commitment of the private sector to philanthropy. This resource will always be vital for renewal of hospital plants, for seed money to initiate new programs, and for medical research. The occasional attempts of regulatory agencies to apply such funds to operating needs are shortsighted. This "quick fix" approach will not yield enough money, and it will destroy the private sector's traditional philanthropic commitment to the non-profit voluntary hospital system.

Second, corporate restructuring of the kind recently carried out by several of the larger hospital complexes and groups of hospitals can provide increased flexibility of operation. In the new structure, the board of the holding company may hold profit-making subsidiaries whose revenues are used to benefit other components, such as the hospital, where a shortfall might have occurred because of inadequate reimbursement for care provided to the indigent. Still experimental, this approach is appealing so long as the organization sticks to health care (e.g., a laboratory service subsidiary). However, one questions the motive when the corporate holding company buys a supermarket, as one such group did recently in the Middle West.

Third, arrangements for a system of stepdown care with nursing homes, chronic care facilities, and elder care programs hold considerable theoretical promise. The organizational structure could follow the holding company model or represent a series of affiliations committed to ensuring the smooth flow of patients through the appropriate level of care.

Fourth, use of a voucher system for Medicare patients has the advantage of combining freedom of choice for the patient with some degree of predictability in determining financial exposure for Medicare. Essential for the success of such a proposal would be the elimination of retrospective cost reimbursement and introduction of a prospective pay schedule for hospitals. In addition, regardless of the financial system ultimately selected, serious consideration should be given to some level of copayment or deductible keyed to income. While such payments by the patient will not have much effect on the overall hospital bill, there is a good chance that patients will become more discriminating in their use of the ambulatory system if they have to pay part of the cost.

Fifth, legislation would provide incentives to states to contract for group coverage for Medicaid eligibles on a risk basis. Because of the variability in Medicaid eligibility, a voucher system is not appropriate, but the success of prepaid at-risk programs in Texas and California suggest that the contractual approach can provide the necessary coverage while limiting liability.

There is no doubt that medical care will continue to grow more costly, and there is no doubt that solving the problem is complex, if not the labor of Sisyphus. In our desire to contain costs, we should not lose sight of our commitment to making high quality, innovative medicine available to all of our citizens. Despite the limitation of resources in the next decade, we need not compromise in our pursuit of this goal. Much can be done to improve the efficiency of the health care system, and new methods of delivering and supporting care can be explored. In this process, the private sector can and should play a major role, and the government should do all it can to get out of the direct administration of the health care system.

14. Response

John W. Colloton

Dr. Sanders has provided us with a good overview of the institutions at risk as we attempt to cope with the increasing health care needs of the elderly and indigent in the period ahead. I think he correctly identifies teaching hospitals and medical schools as institutions in prime jeopardy. Some of you may recall that at this conference last year we quantified the $2 billion of charity care currently being provided by the nation's 270 prime teaching hospitals. That projection was confirmed recently by an American Hospital Association annual survey which showed that the AAMC's Council of Teaching Hospitals, making up only 5.6 percent of the nation's hospitals, incurred $1.8 billion in charity and bad debts during 1980 (table 14.1). This figure, which was approximately 40 percent of the total incurred by all hospitals, averaged $5.4 million per teaching hospital. It should be recognized by all that teaching hospitals, and for that matter all hospitals, can provide such uncompensated care only to some limited and reasonable extent on a continuing basis.

Perhaps at this stage of discussion, my best contribution to an analysis of the institutions at risk would come through describing the specific impact that current and impending cutbacks in the financing of health care for the aged and poor are having in one teaching hospital. In doing so, I will attempt to relate the strategic planning at the University of Iowa Hospitals—a 1,050-bed comprehensive tertiary care center serving the entire state of Iowa—to the possible solutions suggested by Dr. Sanders and others.

We have set all-time records in numbers of admissions in each of the past five years, reaching some 40,000 admissions in 1981 (see figure 14.1).

The clinic operation is growing at the rate of 5 percent each year. Approximately 333,000 clinic visits were recorded in 1981 (figure 14.2).

As table 14.2 shows, our educational mission is embodied in thirty-five

Table 14.1. Charity and bad debts: Council of Teaching Hospitals (COTH) members vs. non-COTH members, 1980

	COTH members	non-COTH members	Total
Numbers of hospitals	327 (5.6%)	5,503 (94.4%)	5,830 (100%)
Bad debts and charity	$1,780,000,000 (38.7%)	$2,820,000,000 (61.3%)	$4,600,000,000 (100%)
Average bad debts charity/hospital	$ 5,443,425	$ 512,447	$ 789,022

Source: American Hospital Association Annual Survey of Hospitals via Council of Teaching Hospitals.

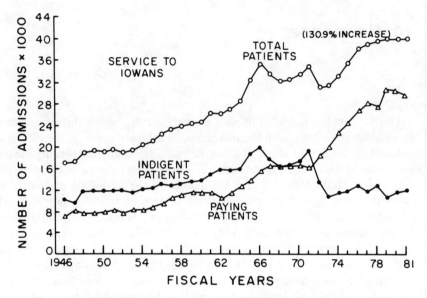

Figure 14.1. Growth in number of admissions by financial classification, University of Iowa Hospitals and Clinics, 1946–81

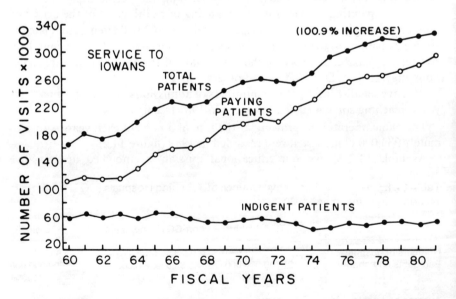

Figure 14.2. Growth in outpatient visits by financial classification, University of Iowa Hospitals and Clinics, FY 1960 through FY 1981

Table 14.2. Health science students training within University of Iowa Hospitals and Clinics

Programs	Number of students
Dentistry and dental hygiene	192
College of nursing	307
Pharmacy residents and undergraduates	63
Physical therapy	63
Hospital and health administration	70
Residents and fellows	542
Medical undergraduates	535
Dietetic interns and graduates	17
Medical technology	29
X-Ray, ultrasound, nuclear medicine, and radiation therapy technology	53
Physician's assistants	38
Respiratory therapy	32
Pastoral service	5
Social service	12
Medical records	2
Speech pathology and audiology	190
Education service interns	8
Occupational therapy interns	2
Activities therapy interns	9
EEG technology students	7
Orthoptist training program	2
Total	2,178

programs that involve almost 2,200 health science collegiate and allied health students.

We sponsor a full array of graduate medical education programs with 542 physicians in training as of 1981–82 (figure 14.3).

Moving on to cost effectiveness, table 14.3 presents the ratio of staff to occupied bed of the nation's sixty-two university-owned hospitals. The University of Iowa Hospitals stands fifth lowest in the nation with a ratio of 4.3 staff members per occupied bed.

In table 14.4 we see a similar comparison of nonpayroll expense per occupied bed among the nation's university-owned teaching hospitals. The University of Iowa Hospitals is in fifty-seventh position among them with an expenditure level of $41,933 per year for each occupied bed.

The comparative average per diem cost among these hospitals is shown in table 14.5. The University of Iowa Hospitals is in fifty-fifth position with an average cost of $240.92 per day.

Figure 14.4 shows us the average length of stay at the University of Iowa Hospitals, which has been reduced from 9.7 days in 1972–73 to 7.8 days as of 1978–79.

Since 1966 we have reduced our number of beds from 1,247 to 1,053, while at the same time increasing the occupancy rate to 83 percent (see figure 14.5).

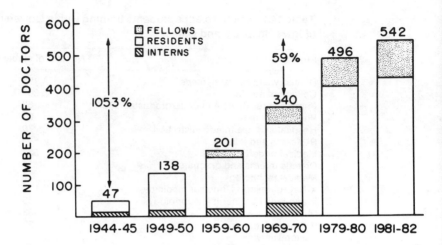

Figure 14.3. Doctors in specialty training, University of Iowa Hospitals and Clinics, FY 1960 through FY 1981

Table 14.3. Number of staff per occupied bed, University of Iowa Hospitals and Clinics, FY 1979

First quartile	Second quartile	Third quartile	Fourth quartile
1. 10.11	17. 6.47	33. 5.36	48. 4.78
2. 8.85	18. 6.28	34. 5.36	49. 4.74
3. 7.74	19. 6.00	35. 5.34	50. 4.68
4. 7.49	20. 5.96	36. 5.34	51. 4.67
5. 7.15	21. 5.95	37. 5.29	52. 4.67
6. 7.05	22. 5.92	38. 5.10	53. 4.59
7. 7.04	23. 5.78	39. 5.08	54. 4.43
8. 7.03	24. 5.72	40. 5.05	55. 4.43
9. 6.86	25. 5.67	41. 5.02	56. 4.42
10. 6.81	26. 5.61	42. 4.99	57. 4.37
11. 6.79	27. 5.58	43. 4.95	58. 4.32
12. 6.77	28. 5.56	44. 4.91	59. 4.26
13. 6.69	29. 5.49	45. 4.79	60. 4.26
14. 6.68	30. 5.47	46. 4.79	61. 3.69
15. 6.53	31. 5.44	47. 4.79	62. 3.37
16. 6.49	32. 5.37		

Table 14.6 presents the rate of hospital use per one thousand Blue Cross members for residents of Johnson County, site of the University of Iowa. In 1981 this rate was 461 days compared to 467 days per one thousand members of HMO plans.

I have set forth all these figures and tables for two purposes. First, to let you know that we have been doing all those things that the so-called powers on high asked us to do. And second, to place the next few tables in context.

Table 14.4. Nonpayroll expense per occupied bed by hospital, University of Iowa Hospitals and Clinics, FY 1979

First quartile		Second quartile		Third quartile		Fourth quartile	
1.	$126,450	17.	$67,364	33.	$56,690	49.	$49,890
2.	122,949	18.	65,708	34.	56,539	50.	49,044
3.	94,344	19.	65,635	35.	56,399	51.	48,609
4.	89,179	20.	65,262	36.	55,677	52.	48,126
5.	85,066	21.	65,013	37.	54,407	53.	48,409
6.	83,400	22.	64,635	38.	53,923	54.	47,014
7.	82,905	23.	64,275	39.	53,598	55.	44,765
8.	75,608	24.	62,807	40.	52,828	56.	42,461
9.	73,702	25.	62,163	41.	52,443	57.	41,933
10.	72,957	26.	60,808	42.	51,328	58.	41,417
11.	72,916	27.	60,568	43.	50,966	59.	38,980
12.	72,196	28.	60,411	44.	50,316	60.	38,391
13.	70,827	29.	58,834	45.	50,070	61.	36,024
14.	68,866	30.	58,405	46.	49,930	62.	34,968
15.	68,166	31.	58,193	47.	49,442	63.	34,838
16.	67,513	32.	56,993	48.	49,215		

Table 14.5. Cost per day for inpatient services by hospital, University of Iowa Hospitals and Clinics, FY 1979

First quartile		Second quartile		Third quartile		Fourth quartile	
1.	$521.22	17.	$353.84	33.	$310.95	49.	$258.84
2.	504.46	18.	351.03	34.	308.97	50.	257.13
3.	503.32	19.	349.47	35.	306.96	51.	249.27
4.	460.93	20.	348.18	36.	304.34	52.	247.20
5.	431.47	21.	343.70	37.	300.97	53.	245.12
6.	416.10	22.	343.20	38.	298.50	54.	243.83
7.	416.10	23.	332.17	39.	295.00	55.	240.92
8.	409.28	24.	331.50	40.	287.19	56.	239.63
9.	397.61	25.	326.84	41.	283.74	57.	235.73
10.	386.66	26.	326.42	42.	280.64	58.	235.28
11.	386.33	27.	325.58	43.	278.66	59.	224.51
12.	386.14	28.	323.44	44.	278.11	60.	198.37
13.	384.31	29.	321.15	45.	276.86	61.	195.47
14.	365.74	30.	319.87	46.	276.85	62.	175.96
15.	362.00	31.	314.72	47.	266.48	63.	168.02
16.	354.40	32.	311.85	48.	264.38		

Table 14.7 portrays our patient census composition, highlighting the aged and indigent components. Next, our 1982–83 reimbursement shortfalls, totaling $13 million, are delineated in table 14.8.

Applying each of Dr. Sanders' suggested solutions, which would be very appropriate for some institutions, would yield little pay dirt in our particular setting. To begin with, we have no problem with clarity of mission or statewide support; we have no marketing problem (as figures 14.1 and 14.2 demonstrate);

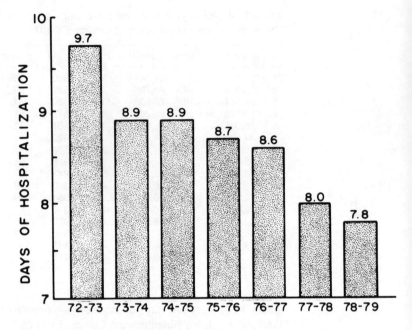

Figure 14.4. Average length of patient stay, University of Iowa Hospitals and Clinics, 1972–73 through 1978–79

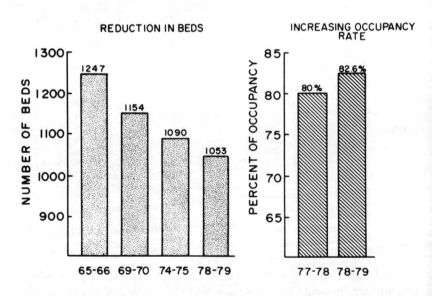

Figure 14.5. Reduction in number of operating beds and increase in occupancy, University of Iowa Hospitals and Clinics, 1965–66 through 1978–79

Table 14.6. Comparison of hospital utilization rates for HMO and Blue Cross members of Johnson County, Iowa, 1981

	Hospital days per 1,000 members
180 prepaid health plans[a]	467
Johnson County, Iowa[b]	
(University of Iowa Hospitals & Clinics)	461

a. U.S. Department of Health and Human Services, *National HMO Census, 1981*, p. 11.
b. Iowa H.S.A., *Comparative Hospital Utilization and Costs*, March 1982.

Table 14.7. Inpatient census composition, University of Iowa Hospitals and Clinics, 1981–82

Aged and indigent patients	
Medicare	25%
Medicaid	7
Iowa's University Hospital Indigent Program	25
Subtotal—aged and indigent patients	57
Other patients	43
Total patients	100%

Table 14.8. Projected payment shortfalls by aged and indigent patient programs, University of Iowa Hospitals and Clinics, 1982–83 (in millions of dollars)

	Current reimbursement formula	Proposed formula revision	Total payment shortfall
Medicare program	$ 4.2	$ 1.1	$ 5.3
Medicaid program	1.1	.2	1.3
Iowa's University Hospital Indigent Patient Care Program	5.3	1.1	6.4
Grand total aged and indigent patient program payment shortfalls	$10.6	$2.4	$13.0[a]

a. Excludes $13.0 million of professional services rendered indigent patients without charge.

and we have little difficulty in limiting the intake of patients to those who can actually be assisted by our services. We are caring for the terminally ill in the traditional manner, which, we believe, is all that can be expected at this juncture. And, finally, for a state university hospital philanthropy is inadequate to solve the shortfall problem. In addition, we have good vertical integration with community physicians, hospitals, and long-term care facilities, so that we are able to move patients through the system in accord with clinical need.

Table 14.9. Proposed short-term solutions to payment shortfalls of aged and indigent patient programs, University of Iowa Hospitals and Clinics, 1982–83 (in millions of dollars)

	Funding source
Subsidy of Medicare, Medicaid, and medically needy patients by other patients and payers	$10.6
Cost containment initiatives	.6
Shift to counties—payment responsibility for indigent patients previously borne by state	1.3
Deferred capital expenditures	.5
Total	$13.0

Accordingly the planned short-term solutions for 1982–83 are several and are portrayed in table 14.9. We plan to cope with 1982–83 shortfalls by taking the following steps:

(*a*) Medicare, Medicaid, and medically needy patients will be subsidized through premium charges to other patients. This practice will generate $10.6 million.

(*b*) We will initiate further cost containment practices that will save some $600,000.

(*c*) Costs of $1.3 million for indigent patients will be transferred from state to county responsibility.

(*d*) Finally, we will defer capital expenditures that total $500,000.

For the long-run solution to this problem we subscribe to the view expressed by Dr. Rogers, Professor Davis, and several others at this conference, namely, that we need to heighten the public's awareness of the benefits derived over the past decade from health care focused on our poor and aged citizens. We hope that this heightened awareness, along with reduced inflation, enhanced national productivity, and economies flowing from multiple reforms now occurring within the health system, will result in adequate dollars being made available to fund the care of these patients on a sound, continuing, and equitable basis. Continued reliance on the short-run solutions I have just quantified for one teaching hospital (and which I should say are the norm for most teaching hospitals—some with premium charges as high as 38 percent) will eventually reach that point where they will jeopardize continued production of the multiple societal contributions currently flowing from academic medical centers. At that juncture, the question before academic centers will be whether care of the 30 to 35 percent of patients generating major shortfalls in payment will be permitted to significantly undermine the quality and scope of the *entire* institution. Because many teaching hospitals will be able to largely perpetuate their tripartite missions by serving the 70 percent of patients who pay the full cost of their service, the dilemma will likely be resolved in favor of preserving the institution's broader roles.

Profound changes in the nature of many teaching hospitals will then take place, including some or all of the following:

— A more constricted role for teaching hospitals in serving the poor, accompanied by a reduction in the size of both ambulatory clinic and inpatient operations, to the extent an offsetting influx of paying patients cannot be attracted.

— Reinstatement of two-class patient care system.

— Reduced opportunities for educational program support by teaching hospitals.

— Diminished quality of care flowing from reduced staffing ratios and a more austere patient care and educational environment.

— Less ability to support clinical research efforts of medical and other health science faculties.

— A diminished capacity to undertake the new technology testing essential to maintaining our system on the frontiers of medical science.

If price competition should prevail as the predominant mechanism for allocating health care dollars, even for the 70 percent of patients now paying the full cost of services, the continued production of societal contributions from teaching hospitals and medical schools will be uneven and unpredictable. Some will flourish, while others may flounder, depending on a host of local circumstances and the reasonableness of alternative support for "educational and research" costs.

In our institution we have been and will continue to work hard to stave off major changes in our missions. At this time we feel confident that the aged and poor of Iowa will be cared for without significant disruption. However, as has been abundantly demonstrated during this conference, the achievement of an equitable and politically acceptable level of financial entitlement for the care of aged and poor on a *national* scale is contingent upon a host of economic, social, clinical, ethical, and political variables which make future predictions hazardous. As I'm sure all of us agree, the goal is one that is worthy of our best collective efforts.

15. Response

John C. Beck

It has been said that a nation is judged by the quality of life that it provides for its elder citizens. There seems to be an impasse in trying to deal with the question of caring well for our elderly. There is little evidence that the various parties concerned with this impasse are really prepared to give or change very much.

Although we are speaking about both the elderly and the poor here, the elderly confront different health and social welfare problems than the poor in the younger age groups. It should also be said that the number of elderly poor in this nation has fallen progressively since the early 1960s; if one uses the federal government's definition for the poverty level, the poor now include about 14 percent elderly in contrast to over 20 percent in the 1960s. However, there is a large group of elderly who are near poverty, and they might well be driven into poverty by some of the devices that have been suggested as methods of dealing with their health care.

My colleagues and I are trying to face this situation on a state level in California, and we realize the enormous difficulty of trying to conceive possible solutions. At the same time, we are trying to create educational programs throughout the medical educational continuum, at a time when resources are constrained. And, finally, we are concerned with the creation of new service programs in the academic medical center and in ambulatory sites where the university has never been, such as community sites, sheltered housing facilities, and nursing homes.

The major issue that confronts us is how to provide health care to the elderly at an acceptable cost. There is no question but that demand is going to exceed supply, and some of the very important moral and ethical issues that surfaced very briefly early in our discussion really need to be addressed in great seriousness. I think they are very different from some of the moral and ethical issues that confront us as physicians treating people below the age of sixty-five.

The second thing that I wanted to emphasize is the patient backup actually occurring in our acute hospital system. We thought that there was substantial backup in the West Los Angeles area, but when we began to look at PSRO data tapes we found that, although it was there, it was not as large as expected. At the moment we are looking at a whole series of PSRO data tapes from various parts of the nation to determine how large the problem is.

One thing that many of us who attend the elderly are confronted with, at least in California, is a massive influx of elderly patients from private physicians to university-sponsored activities. When the difference in pay between Medicare and the usual and customary fee made up by MediCal was eliminated, an influx began, and it has been impossible for us to deal with, given our constraints of resources and faculty.

The dollar flow for services rendered to the elderly by physicians and other health professionals is not adequate to maintain this kind of activity because it is labor intensive and the reimbursement rates are not equivalent to those one would receive for specialized procedures. If that problem is not addressed on a national scale, at some future time we will be in very serious difficulty indeed.

I also wanted to comment about the importance of defining the institution's role. During my last five years with a Canadian institution, prospective budgeting became a reality and led to one extremely useful activity. The board of trustees, the administrative officers, and the professional staff of the institution together identified the institution's mission and, in the process of prospective budgeting, identified which programs they really wanted to see succeed and which ones they were prepared to abandon. That exercise was extremely valuable, and it led to great benefit.

The issue of discharge planning is a critical one. We have been looking at discharge planning in a variety of counties in Southern California, and we have found to our amazement that discharge planning is not really done. We are attempting to utilize our health professionals to educate hospitals in the importance of discharge planning. The only really elegant study of home care services is "The Effects and Costs of Day Care Services for the Chronically Ill," by William Weissert, Thomas Wan, Barbara Livieratos, and Sidney Katz, which appeared in *Medical Care* 18 (1980): 567–84. It suggests that home care services may cost as much as institutional care, if opportunity costs are counted.

At the moment the median age of nursing home residents is eighty-one years; 26 percent of all individuals in this country over the age of eighty-five are actually in nursing homes. At least 26 percent of people over sixty-five will spend some time, not necessarily their terminal time, in a nursing home facility. We know very little about the dynamics of this flow of nursing home patients. Early evidence shows that there clearly are two streams of residents: the so-called slow stream, and a much more rapid stream, for whom the average stay is about three months. We ought not to forget this dynamism when we talk about nursing homes.

Some of my colleagues have been looking at some of the very common problems in nursing homes, one of which is the issue of incontinence. Incontinence accounts for one-third of the cost of nursing home care in the United States. We have found that the prevalence of this disorder, which is highly disabling both from the medical and the social point of view, is really unknown, but it is clearly very high. In our survey of a series of nursing homes in Los Angeles, we found that around 40 to 50 percent of the patients were incontinent. The vast majority of those patients had not had a urinalysis, and less than one percent of them had had any appropriate urological investigation. There are probably a whole series of causes that could be identified, and we are taking steps to understand those. In many instances, appropriate intervention might reverse the disorder and thus reduce costs.

Similarly, a National Center for Health Services Research survey in nursing homes in 1977 reported that between 50 and 70 percent of the residents of nursing homes were intellectually impaired. The vast majority of those individuals had not had the simplest screening procedures to identify those who might have a reversible intellectual impairment, such as an unrecognized depression.

The other thing that I would like to talk about very briefly is our evidence on the quality of care that we, as physicians, deliver to the elderly in this nation. I suspect that we will need not less but more physicians and other health professionals if we are to increase the number of individuals in the so-called fast stream.

Several years ago my colleagues and I looked at physician/patient encounters with a clear bias that the older the patient, the longer the encounter time with the physician would be. Using national data, we discovered that physician/patient encounter time actually decreased with age. In averaging hospital and nonhospital data there was a shortening from 15.3 to 13.7 minutes in the average duration of visits. Simply to make the physician/patient encounter time equivalent to what the rest of the population was receiving, we would need an increase in manpower of somewhere around 12 percent.

Another interesting bit of data is the number of physicians in this country with a commitment to the care of the elderly. In examining the AMA's 1977 data base we found only 629 physicians who considered the care of the elderly their primary, secondary, or tertiary interest. With an 88 percent response rate, this would be roughly 715 out of 363,000 physicians.

A third bit of evidence has to do with the geriatric assessment or evaluation units that are growing up in this country. They all show that, in the elderly population discharged from our acute tertiary care academic institutions, there are three to four unrecognized problems that have not been identified or, if identified, not been dealt with. Dealing with these problems can often make the difference between discharging a patient to the community and discharging to a long-term care institution.

A bit of evidence about the quality of care to our elderly population shows that the 11 percent of the individuals in this nation over the age of sixty-five are utilizing somewhere between 25 to 30 percent of all the prescription drugs that are being sold. One does not have to work with the elderly very long before one realizes that there is inappropriate use of drugs. Not infrequently we see an elderly person who complains of intellectual impairment and takes between twelve and twenty different medications.

I cite these bits of data to show that the quality of care that we are presently delivering to the elderly is not ideal. When we think of the utilization of health services in the future, we may well have to think in terms of more appropriate services to that population. One of the major constraints on solving the problem is the inadequate number of appropriately trained health professionals in this

area: physicians, nurses, social workers, pharmacists, occupational physiothera-
pists, and so forth.

A year or two ago we predicted that this nation needed a minimum of 900
faculty members in medicine and family practice and 450 in gero-psychiatry
simply to begin to improve the quality of our physician educational performance. We also predicted that by 1990 this nation would need 7,000 to 10,000
full-time equivalent physicians to look after the elderly population. That pre-
diction was based on some pretty firm assumptions, particularly the utilization
rates of physician services among the elderly and a substantial delegation of
responsibilities for the care of the elderly to such physician extenders as physician assistants and nurse practitioners. There is a tremendous challenge to this
nation to redirect some of the potential physician excess into care for the elderly,
to improve our knowledge in the area, and to make more economical use of
health services.

And finally, I want to emphasize the importance of research. The National
Institute of Aging has attempted through its short history to stimulate the production of research faculty for the health professional schools. There are very
few physicians and nurses in that population, yet some of these issues have to be
addressed by health professionals trained in research, and there are practically
none. If we are really to get at issues of importance in the long-term care system,
such as intellectual impairment or incontinence, we will need research support.

Discussion

Dr. Wilbur: I gather from Dr. Sanders' and Mr. Colloton's remarks that academic health centers cannot continue doing as they have done in the past. Either the university centers must become the institutions of last resort for the aged and the poor, as the public institutions were in the past but probably can no longer be in the future, or else they must become tertiary care institutions devoted to relatively cost ineffective, highly specialized services, such as burn units, that are needed infrequently but are indispensable when they are needed.

One of the other sources of support for academic health centers is the use of the faculty in private research supported by pharmaceutical companies or other private institutions. In fact, the support of the academic centers in the future may include corporate restructuring to enable clinical faculty to become involved in gene splicing or some other attractive research area to help support the institution.

We need some ideas as to which directions the various university centers will have to go, about how successful or how safe the idea of making arrangements with private industry will be, and whether this will totally change the academic health centers from anything we have known in the past.

Mr. MacNaughton: Dr. Sanders used the phrase "cream skimmers" in connection with the for-profit hospital groups, a phrase I think is rather meaningless. Let me respond for the Hospital Corporation of America to the accusation that we skim the cream. In 152 of the communities in which we own hospitals or manage them for others, ours is the only hospital. It is our company policy to accept into those hospitals anybody who comes to them, including all the indigents in the community. Most of these are small communities, but they have their share of indigents.

In cities where we have competition for our business, it is our company policy to take our fair share of the medically indigent. Besides caring for them without fee, we also assumed in 1980, for example, bad debts that amounted to $25 million. Those indigents who required tertiary care were referred to teaching hospitals. In locations where we are beginning to develop tertiary care centers, we try to take care of them ourselves.

I would also like to amplify a comment that Dr. Sanders made about the fact that Prudential Insurance Company announced at the end of last year that it was going to stop selling individual health insurance policies. At the beginning of last year Prudential did what it always does. It built into its premium structure the medical inflation rate anticipated for the year 1981, and the assumptions were fine until about the middle of the year. All of a sudden, the curve shot straight up, and it continued straight up for the next two quarters, at which time Prudential announced the cessation of sales of new individual policies. Part of the problem Prudential has run into may result from the fact that when insurers sell individual insurance policies they develop a block of business, the top of which contains the best risk and the bottom of which contains the poorest risk. Every time they have to raise the rate to correct for inflation, they lose a little bit of the block at the top. Eventually, those who remain are all bad risk: people who are going to be sick or who are sick. When that is the case, the curve shoots straight up and that might well be what happened to Prudential in 1981, and I daresay if it happened to Prudential, it could well happen to any carrier.

Dr. Ellwood: Blue Cross lost almost a million dollars last year in assets. My impression is that several of the other large companies are experiencing this same problem. One of the reasons why we are seeing so many insurers moving to prepayment plans is really not because that is such great business, but because it may be the only business left. I really think we are faced with the disintegration not only of health care for the poor but also of private insurance. I suspect we are seeing it begin to come apart at the seams, and we are facing some very serious problems.

Dr. Hamburg: It seems to me that there are two principal factors that will transform health care over the next few decades. One is the economic factor, about which we have had lengthy discussions, and the other is scientific development, about which we have had very little to say. We are living in a period of absolutely unprecedented development in the life sciences, and it would be tragic if that development were not effectively applied to the problems of the elderly, especially in light of the demographic changes in our population in the next few decades. Besides the surge in molecular and cellular biology, there are significant gains in other aspects of biology, in epidemiology and biostatistics, and in computer technology that have helped population sciences as well as behavioral sciences. How can these impressive developments be focused appropriately on the aging of our population?

Among the crucial targets that can be identified is major memory loss in the elderly. This is a common and severe problem in otherwise reasonably healthy people. Although there has been remarkable progress in the last five years on the neurobiology of memory, very little connection has been made between that basic research and the memory deficits of the elderly. Is there any connection? How can we find out? Are all possible steps being taken by government, by industry, and by academia? This kind of research is not intended to be a quest for eternal life, but rather an improvement in the quality for the natural life span of our species.

The private sector could do a lot in a direct support role, particularly industry. There is also a role for the private sector in using its powerful influence with federal and state governments to support research in this sphere.

I want to say just a quick word about linking voluntary efforts to the practical management of problems of the elderly in communities. Central to this issue is the aim of fostering as much functional independence and personal dignity of the elderly as is possible, and here the role of social support networks is very important. I do not mean support in the economic sense but in the sense of mediating the effects of stress both in promoting health and in responding to illness. That is a major need of the elderly, whether they become institutionalized or not.

There is a body of rather recent research on social support networks showing that they can have a number of protective effects. For example, one study shows that social support networks can reduce psychological distress and physiological abnormalities following job loss or bereavement. There are other studies on protection against emotional problems associated with aging and on promoting adherence to therapeutic regimens through effective social support networks.

Most older people want to live alone, but there are limitations. Many of these limitations, involving transportation, shopping, companionship, organizing daily tasks, could be offset without heroic efforts or heavy expense. An important question, though, is the extent to which volunteers can help. There is a lot of informed volunteer help in our communities now, but it probably could be augmented by organizing at the neighborhood or community level.

One interesting locus is in the contact between adolescents or young adults and old people. Adolescents and young adults are very seriously looking for a useful role. Many of them feel, at least privately, rather lost and useless; on the other hand, older people need the kind of practical help that young people could provide. How can you connect willing and able young people with older people who need their help? Possibly through senior high schools and colleges, through work sites, through the media, through community organizations (especially churches), through hospitals, unions, and co-ops. Emerging community coalitions ought to try to foster effective social networks for the elderly in their community with a strong volunteer component.

I want to close with a comment about the upshot of scientific progress. Suppose it really goes well. Suppose science is not seriously eroded in the next couple of decades. Then what? The best scenario, the most attractive one, has been eloquently expressed by Lewis Thomas: "With greater understanding of biological mechanisms and with a decrease in health damaging behavior, we could get to the point where most people would live vigorous lives, and then pass quietly in the night when their biological clocks run out."

Until that great day arrives, however, we are going to have to deal with the problem of costs. The more successful we are in promoting vigorous life through the midseventies, the more we will increase the most rapidly growing segment of our population, the group above seventy-five, which uses the most health care services.

Dr. Estes: The personal care that the elderly require is highly labor intensive. This is an ideal area for the heavy and cost effective utilization of mid-level practitioners, such as nurse practitioners and physician assistants, and yet Medicare has not been willing to pay for those services under Part B because the Medicare law was written before PAs and nurse practitioners were well established and such services were not anticipated. The law is written very specifically: Part B will only pay for physicians' services and those services directly flowing from their activities, such as injections, dressings, etc. This is an area in which a policy change could be very cost efficient down the road.

Dr. Ellwood: If we are going to be dealing with a population that is aging with a variety of long-term complaints, then the economic and the social responsibility for these people has to be extended. Wouldn't the problems of the University of Iowa Hospitals be solved if they were paid on a per capita basis? As John Colloton showed, that is a comprehensive, efficient health system, but it is trapped by the squeeze on unit prices. The hospital utilization rate in Johnson County, Iowa, is 462 days per thousand, which would make it one of the lowest hospital utilization rates in the United States. In Des Moines, the utilization rate is 2100 per thousand, the highest utilization in the state. It seems to me that the university should be rewarded for its efficiency and one way would be to pay it in a different way, at a rate based on the average for the state, for example.

Dr. David Rogers: We are extending life, and people might argue that we are simply going to continue to balloon the cost of health care for the elderly. The fact that we have more and more elderly does not inevitably mean that we are going to have horrendously increasing health care costs.

Dr. Sanders mentioned that he thought universities were beginning to try to dissociate themselves from their teaching hospitals. My recent observations indicate precisely the opposite. I find that teaching hospitals, under enormous constraints and the pressures of the regulatory apparatus, are saying, "We don't want that medical school. We don't want to have students messing up the place and costing us all that money. We don't want to support Fellows. We would really prefer that you go away." This worries me enormously. The strength of our whole medical enterprise has been the wedding of a hospital to a teaching unit, and now I see them trying to divorce one another. But I find that it is the hospital that is trying to divorce the university, not the other way around.

Dr. Nelson: I wanted to ask Mr. Etheredge about the capacity of the Veterans Administration program to help with some of the problems that we have been discussing here.

Mr. Etheredge: I think there is a very large potential. Within the next ten years about 60 percent of the male population over sixty-five will be veterans. Under current law as soon as veterans become sixty-five, they are deemed to be service disabled and therefore have a right to free care at veterans' facilities. There will thus be tremendous pressure on the whole veterans' system. It is already the largest long-term care provider in the country, and it is going to become even more important as a long-term care provider over the next decade. Most of the beds in veterans' hospitals are now filled with nonservice disabled people, so there is reserve capacity to meet these needs.

Another aspect of the question is the affiliation of veterans' hospitals with universities. That relationship has always been one of the great strengths of the system, and I think the Veterans Administration wants to continue it. The future growth of the Veterans Administration services will be in long-term rather than acute care; whether medical schools are interested in shifting their training programs to match these VA needs is a question that is still unresolved.

Dr. Ginzberg: I would like to try to link a couple of themes that have emerged in discussion during the last two days.

It is clear, whether we like it or not, that both the federal and state governments are trying in many different ways to reduce, or to slow the rate of increase in, their expenditures for health care. So far, that effort has not endangered the system because of the capacity to shift part of the reduction to other payers. We have had considerable discussion of the next consequence of that reduction, which will be a diminution in services, and that is likely to have adverse effects on people with less money. We have tried to identify the critical actors operating in this very open and complicated system, and we have listed the government, the insurance companies, the academic health centers, and hospitals in general.

The next question is: How much possibility is there for any significant response by these other actors, given the fact that the government controls 40 percent of the total dollars. We don't think that the academic health centers have an easy way of generating response money. Many of the hospitals with a large exposure to the poor or to patients who are only partially subsidized are going to be in trouble. It looks as if the insurance business is also going to be in trouble.

We have survived for years in a very loose system because the monies were flowing pretty freely. Since individual actions will have little impact on the situation we are now facing, the question is: What are the possibilities of *collective* action? Business coalitions are one possibility for the future, but it will take a while to put them in place. Wherever there are multiple academic health centers, there is some scope for a collective response to their situation, although they don't know it yet, and they move very slowly.

I think that the market impact on hospitals will be quite effective, although it may not have the effect one would like. I think we are going to see a large number of closures, mergers, disappearances, and reductions in capacity. In general, this is a move in the right direction, but it leaves some exposed population groups. That is what we must keep watching.

There is no question that we ought to move as self-consciously as possible to instruments of collective action, among which prospective budgeting is the outstanding one. We will have to get some system of socializing the unpaid costs of health care for the poor and aged, perhaps some form of business coalition. We are surely not going to let people disappear from the care system, so the question really is whether we use our time to get slightly better resolutions in a difficult world, or whether we fail to take the time that we have and then are forced into worse decisions later on.

Dr. Ellwood: I am troubled by the notion of dealing with this through socialization of costs. I am convinced that we spend enough on medical care. The data out of Rochester, Minnesota, and Johnson County, Iowa, indicate that people get superb medical care on much less hospitalization than the average in the country. Do we really need to spend as much on hospitalization as we do? Do we have a problem of too much money being spent on the wrong thing, or do we have a problem of not spending enough money on the poor? I think it is not a matter of cost subsidies; it is a matter of eliminating waste.

Mr. Onek: I was struck by Mr. MacNaughton's description of the Prudential problem as he sees it: a large block of insured people, with a significant number of bad risks. I wonder where the good risks went. I assume they went to another insurance company. It strikes me that the problem that the Prudential and Blue Cross are facing is directly parallel to the problem that the tertiary care centers are facing. When you have only one insurance company, there can be a great deal of cross subsidization and you do not have a problem. If there is only one hospital in the community and it provides primary, secondary, and tertiary care, there can also be a great deal of cross subsidization. But as soon as you segment the market, which we have done by having a system with a great many insurance companies and different types of hospitals, cross subsidization ceases. The problem then becomes one of survival in a world where for a variety of reasons there is going to be a great deal less cross subsidization. The institutions that used to live by that kind of cross subsidization have a new task: to get subsidized more openly and more directly by government or philanthropic sources and to justify their need for that direct subsidization. The only alternative is the mass cross subsidization of a national health program.

Prof. Reinhardt: Basically, the gist of this conference is that we're in one hell of a fix or sliding into it fast. Our goal is to produce, distribute, and finance health care. There are two principles you could use to do this. One is solidarity: if you break your leg, the medical care you recieve is totally independent of your income and socioeconomic status. It does not necessarily mean that the treatment will be the same everywhere in the country, but what happens to you when you break your leg is no longer a function of your income. That's solidarity. The alternative is a two-tier, or multi-tier, health care system where we will guarantee the poor something, which we will discuss openly, and the rest of the people pay for themselves.

It is my feeling, after living here a decade or more, that solidarity is not the sort of thing Americans like. Now, this is odd, especially because physicians practice solidarity, by and large, within the confines of their practice. Once patients come through the door, physicians treat them regardless of economic status. Yet physicians have always used their political power to prevent the very establishment of the system that could bring solidarity into the health care system.

Maybe the time has come for a two-tier system. England has one, and so does West Germany. We would need to accept the two-tier system as a principle, not just as an undesirable outcome, and then we could discuss the quality of the bottom tier.

A survey has just been completed by the *New York Times* and CBS. It included this question: "If it would reduce the cost of health care, would you be willing to go to a clinic where you would be assigned an available doctor instead of going to see your own private doctor?" Fifty percent of the respondents answered "Yes"; they would be willing to have limited choice if it would reduce costs. Another question: "If it would reduce the cost of health care, would you be willing to have your routine illnesses treated by a nurse or a doctor's assistant rather than by a doctor?" And 58 percent of the people said "Yes."

Conceivably, when we think of solutions we might ask the people what they want, rather than asking the professionals what they think the people ought to have. Maybe limiting choice for some people is the ultimate solution. If we were to go the two-tier route, what should the bottom package be? Maybe one would go the HMO route in the end and let the people who want unlimited choice pay for it out of their own pockets.

Dr. Sanders: First of all, I think the private insurers are in serious trouble. The difficulty is not unique to the Blues; it affects all fiscal intermediaries. If I were forecasting a 20 percent premium to subsidize my shortfall over the next couple of years on the basis of commercial insurance, I would not feel a great deal of confidence.

The second point I would make is that, while it is true that the dollar flow to the physician extenders does not meet the need, I do not think that the dollar numbers are going to get any greater. It is instead a question of rearrangement and redistribution. That is going to be a very tough issue. I do not quite know how to get from here to there.

I feel very strongly that there is a place for HMOs and a place for proprietaries, a place for the nonprofit hospitals, and a place for the public hospitals. The thing that seems to be in greatest jeopardy as we economize, even in university hospitals, is the training of people, be they physicians or paramedical personnel. Trying to deliver a large amount of care in the shortest possible time does not necessarily mean that we are preparing ourselves to take care of the challenges of people, and I am very concerned about how we meet those challenges. I think it can be done, but we have to recognize what we are doing to ourselves in the process.

As far as Dr. Wilbur's comments are concerned, I really did not talk about restructuring business. For those medical centers that are large enough, there is no reason why you cannot make contractual arrangements with other facilities to provide services, resulting in a laboratory organization that can provide some margin of profitability. That is the American way of life. For those who are innovative, I am sure a lot can be done, but it does go against some of the usual traditions of the nonprofit sector. I think we ought to get over that problem.

Let me speak very briefly about the term "skimming." If you are a publicly held company, hospital, or corporation, you have to be pretty sound in your business decisions as to what kind of communities you are going to enter, what the return on your investment is going to be, how much free care you are willing to accept, and how much you are willing to put back into the system in terms of education. I don't think that proprietary hospitals are either very interested in or capable of educating young physicians.

In response to Dr. Rogers' comment about the hospitals trying to divorce the universities, I agree that there is a bit of that. I think there is going to be continuing tension between the hospital and other elements of the university that is going to have to be sorted out. It may result in a restructuring of the way things are done, but nevertheless I do not think it can be allowed to continue if the essence of the university atmosphere is to be maintained. I think they can coexist nervously, at least for awhile. Research is absolutely essential. We do not pay nearly enough attention to research, and it is one area where many of the solutions will be found.

Finally, I do not think anything is going to happen until the shoe really begins to pinch the reimbursement foot. Prospective reimbursement seems to be attractive. We have been talking about it for years, but we have not done anything about it. We are getting to the point, however, where financial limitations are going to force us to restructure the reimbursement system. Once that happens, behavioral modifications will result in all kinds of innovative structures.

Chairman Anlyan: On that hopeful note, let us close. Thank you all for coming.

Index